A Great Literature Guide to the DSM-5®

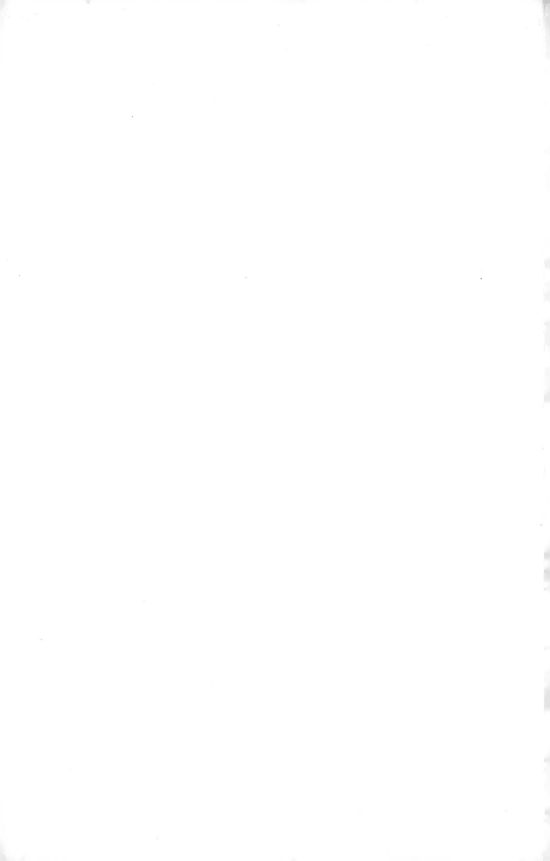

A Great Literature Guide to the

❧ DSM-5® ❧

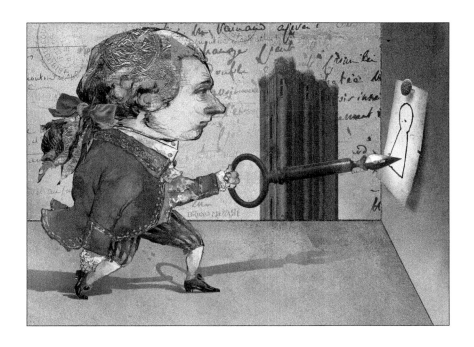

Eric L. Altschuler, M.D., Ph.D

Metropolitan Hospital, New York City

About the Cover
Image © Bruno Mallart
Bruno Mallart is one of the most talented European artists, his work having appeared in some of the world's premier publications: *The New York Times, The Wall Street Journal,* and the *New Scientist,* to name a few. A freelance illustrator since 1986, Mallart first worked for several children's book publishers and advertising agencies, using a classical realistic watercolor and ink style. Some years later he began working in a more imaginative way, inventing a mix of drawing, painting, and collage. His work speaks of a surrealistic and absurd world and engages the viewer's imagination and sense of fun. Despite the recurring use of the brain in his art, Mallart's background is not scientific—though his parents were both neurobiologists. He uses the brain as a symbol for abstract concepts such as intelligence, thinking, feeling, ideas, and knowledge. Attracted to all that is mechanical, Mallart's art frequently includes machine parts such as gears and wheels that imply movement and rhythm. To see more of Bruno Mallart's art, please go to his website: www.brunomallart.com.

Oxford University Press is a department of the University of Oxford. It furthers the University's objective of excellence in research, scholarship, and education by publishing worldwide. Oxford is a registered trade mark of Oxford University Press in the UK and certain other countries.

Published in the United States of America by Oxford University Press
198 Madison Avenue, New York, NY 10016, United States of America

A Great Literature Guide to the DSM-5®
© 2018 Oxford University Press
Sinauer Associates is an imprint of Oxford University Press.

For titles covered by Section 112 of the US Higher Education Opportunity Act, please visit www.oup.com/us/he for the latest information about pricing and alternate formats.

Address editorial correspondence to:
Sinauer Associates
P.O. Box 407
Sunderland, MA 01375 U.S.A.
publish@sinauer.com

Address orders, sales, license, permissions, and translation inquiries to:
Oxford University Press U.S.A.
2001 Evans Road
Cary, NC 27513 U.S.A.
Orders: 1-800-445-9714

Library of Congress Cataloging-in-Publication Data
Names: Altschuler, Eric Lewin, author.
Title: A great literature guide to the DSM-5 / Eric L. Altschuler.
Description: Sunderland, Massachusetts : Sinauer Associates, Inc. Publishers, 2017.
Identifiers: LCCN 2017003679 | ISBN 9781605356761 (pbk.)
Subjects: LCSH: Mental illness in literature. | Diseases in literature. |
   Characters and characteristics in literature. | Psychology and literature.
   | Diagnostic and statistical manual of mental disorders. 5th ed

Classification: LCC PN56.M45 A47 2017 | DDC 809/.93353--dc23
LC record available at https://lccn.loc.gov/2017003679

9 8 7 6 5 4 3 2 1
Printed in the United States of America

*Bettina and I thank Benjamin and Daniel.
We have discussed many of the stories and
tales herein. Many more. L'dor vador.*

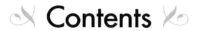 Contents

Preface

One of the many delights of being in medical research—especially basic or "pure" research is that one gets to retreat from the "real world" with all its limitations and mind-numbing social arbitrariness. And one of the perks is the opportunity to interact with a wide range of exceptionally creative minds. I have had the good fortune of surrounding myself with many colorfully eccentric and brilliant colleagues and students. Eric Altschuler is very near the top of my list in terms of the breadth of his interests and passionate involvement in research. When he joined my lab as a medical student, he had already published a book on the composer J. S. Bach and a paper in *Physical Review Letters*. We have and continue to collaborate on a number of studies using mirror visual feedback as a tool to enable or accelerate recovery from stroke paralysis, hemispatial neglect, and phantom limb pain. After his stint in my lab Dr. Altschuler has as a physician and researcher initiated several new lines of inquiry and become world-renowned for changing our perspective on neuro-rehabilitation.

Anyone who has the good fortune to run into Eric cannot fail to notice his contagious enthusiasm and his ability to see medical research as a grand unfolding adventure punctuated by landmark discoveries. This makes him a very effective teacher and expositor. He makes otherwise drab narratives about diseases come to life by placing them in proper historical context. This book is full of such examples and I hope it will become prescribed reading just like the books of Lewis Thomas, Berton Roueché, and Paul De Kruif. Reading about such discoveries and hidden connections makes you feel like medical research is a great party which you are being invited to join.

One day Eric and I were looking around the UCSD Bookstore and he called me over and said, "Rama, they've started a new section on the history of neuroscience." I responded that we are living the history of neuroscience. So many questions from the 20th, 19th, even 18th century are still relevant today.

Curiously and remarkably, Eric has found that when studying psychiatric disease one can go much further back in time, many centuries, even many millennia and find in great literature—Shakespeare, Homer, the Bible—almost complete descriptions of the diseases!

Eric's approach of using "cases" from great literature to illustrate and guide the learner through the DSM-5® is ingenious and should be of great benefit to students at all levels (and their teachers). The authors of the classics somehow seem to have had an advance copy of DSM-5 long before it was even written and the diseases are vividly described once one appreciates that they are there—as shown us by Eric. He notes that while the cases of DSM-5 diseases found in great literature can be seen as surprisingly informative "sketches" of the diagnoses, they are much more. In all instances, the plot thickens and more and more information about a disease or condition emerges year-by-year. This progressive detective work that leads to understanding would serve the valuable purpose of stimulating the curiosity of students, physicians, psychologists, mental and other healthcare personnel, researchers, as well as patients and their families. We get to see glimpses of "director's cuts" of the DSM-5 and the diseases it covers much of which is still not fully understood or appreciated today.

The deep insight that the Bard had into the human condition—whether in health or disease—can be illustrated with two of my favorite examples, both from Macbeth. In one passage Shakespeare anticipates much of Freudian psychoanalysis and the power of the unconscious:

[Doctor] Cure her of that.

Canst thou not minister to a mind diseased,

Pluck from the memory a rooted sorrow,

Raze out the written troubles of the brain

And with some sweet oblivious antidote

Cleanse the stuffed bosom of that perilous stuff

Which weighs upon the heart?

Elsewhere, her Ladyship clearly displays OCD traits as she sleepwalks to the basin, washing her hands repeatedly to metaphorically wash away her sin—the murder of Duncan. Yet, "All the perfumes of Arabia will not sweeten this little hand." Note that this isn't merely the contamination-aversion (e.g., after touching door knobs) and ritual hand washing which characterizes OCD but *metaphorically* washing away *moral* contamination (from having committed murder) so the contamination itself is metaphorical rather than literal. In this one line the Bard anticipates much of what has been called "embodied cognition"—that even so-called abstract ideation is powerfully anchored in—and constrained by the physical flesh of the body and its movements.

No doubt inspired by this book, readers will find new examples of psychiatric and neuropsychiatric diseases. When you do, please send them to Eric and me. We want to hear about them!

Acknowledgments

I thank my teachers for firing an interest in history and its utility. In Ms. Takousian's fifth-grade class, where math and science were Greek geometry proofs and Egyptian and medieval construction methods, English was *Detectives in Togas*, social studies went from the Nile through the 116 years of the Hundred Years War. I'd also like to thank: Orley Samuels, Ms. Kay, Mrs. Huback (Principal), Mr. Sug, Ms. Elfant, Simcha Rosenberg, Ms. Finnegan, Simcha Weintraub, Ms. Cohen, Joey Garen-Wolf, John Ruskay (Principal), Cantor Kornreich, Rabbi Alan Miller, Ms. Goddell, Mr. Livingstone, Mr. Shedlan (Principal), Ms. Kathryn Brainard, Mr. Robert Sharon, Madame Spodheim, Mrs. Ellis, Ms. Burt, Mr. Zimbalist, Mrs. Sterbenz, Mr. Gold, Mr. Hubner, Professor Tom Benjamin, Mr. Geller, Mr. Ritterman, Mrs. Dahlberg, Mr. Micklow, Mr. Kramer, Mr. Bindman, Ms. Cantor, Dr. Jamo Blake, Dr. Rothenberg, Mr. Rutkowski, Mr. Watras, Mr. Murray Kahn (Assistant Principal), Mr. Lehrman (Assistant Principal), Mr. Abraham Baumel (Principal), Mr. Matta (Assistant Coach), Mr. Fitzpatrick (Assistant Coach), Assistant Coach Velkas, Assistant Coach Hahn, Coach Blaufarb, Professor Calvert Watkins, Professor Stephen Jay Gould, Professor Andrew M. Gleason, Professor Frederick Wooten, Dr. Farid Dowla, Dr. Masoud Seyal, Dr. Albert Ray, Dr. John Grimaldi, Professor VS Ramachandran, MD, PhD, Dr. Amar Butt, Dr. Adam Stein, Dr. Jerry Weissman, Dr. David Bressler, Dr. Kristjan Ragnarsson (Chair), Dr. Joel DeLisa (Chair). And my students, residents, colleagues, and patients.

I thank my mother, Sheila Brody. She encouraged my interest in "applied literature." She also read through the *Iliad* and the *Odyssey* looking for hints and traces of literature predating Homer's epics.

I would like to thank my editor extraordinaire, Sydney Carroll. It's harder to edit a book than to write it, because you need to end up with the same product, but work with/through the writer to get this accomplished! Not only did this book improve with each round of editing corrections, but each time Sydney's comments led me to add important information or refine the logic or understanding of a subject. When this book started I had a collection of papers about psychiatric disease in literary characters that I had written or written by others that I had found. Due to Sydney's outstanding work, a veritable "DSM-Great Literature" is found to be there in the literature and is now presented here! I would also like to thank Andy Sinauer for his support.

Introduction

THIS BOOK EXAMINES PROMINENT individuals from great literature, mostly protagonists and a few bit players, their apparent mental disorder or disease, how those disorders and diseases meet the DSM-5® (Diagnostic and Statistical Manual-5) diagnostic criteria, and how the authors of these stories could possibly have had enough insight and knowledge to create characters who were so clearly suffering from mental illness hundreds of years before these illnesses were even classified or defined.

But before digging into the diseased minds of figures in great literature, one could wonder how modern readers might dare diagnose characters from great literature and historical figures, even the Bible. Nobel Prize Laureate in Physics Richard Feynman (1918–1988) pointed out that often lay individuals can know as much as or more about a given disease than physicians, because doctors must learn about *all* diseases, while a non-doctor may only have an intense interest in one disease. Thus, by focusing on the method of using the history and some other signs and clues to make a diagnosis, and by looking for them in great literature by astute, observational authors, we might become expert practitioners in this new "undiscovered" aspect of medicine.

Feynman also had a simple rule he used to decide if a given theory or discovery was correct and important. Such discoveries had to have what Feynman called, "the simplicity we typically associate with truth." This beautiful, truthful simplicity is present in an undiscovered undercurrent of exacting and ahead-of-its time descriptions of disease in the Bible and other great literary works throughout history.

How Do Doctors Make a Diagnosis?

Medical diagnosis—finding out any of the millions of ways that the body inevitably betrays us, breaks down and malfunctions—can be a difficult, complex task. And that's just for the physical ailments; the psychiatric maladies are a completely different, and relatively new, frontier.

The doctor really is a detective of sorts. She or he listens to the patient's complaints and problems and systematically, by the information and history provided, tries to fit the clues together so they point toward a particular disease—and often the best remedy. The patient history is supposed to give a doctor a full 80% of the diagnosis. Then, *based on this history*, a physical examination of the patient should be able to provide another 10% of the way to the diagnosis, and then, *based on the history and physical examination*, diagnostics such as blood tests, X-rays, CAT scans, biopsies, etc., should give the last 10% of the diagnosis.

But, psychiatric disease can reside all in the mind. With strictly physical maladies, good doctors don't just skip ahead to the blood test or an MRI—but it sure can be handy. When it comes to psychiatry, a doctor can't just order a blood test to definitively see if a patient has depression, the way an X-ray would show if a bone was broken. In psychiatric disease, the history is perhaps even more important than in diagnosing other kinds of disease, though blood tests, X-rays etc., can be crucial confirmations to make sure that some other process is not causing or contributing to the patient's psychiatric problems.

A strict method underpins forays into the mind, of course. Psychiatric diagnosis is made using the *Diagnostic and Statistical Manual*, or DSM (in its Fifth Edition, the DSM is named DSM-5).

The DSM and Its History

Psychiatry may seem to be the most personal—close to the soul, even—of all medical undertakings. And it may seem paradoxical to use a statistical, methodical manual to delve into this seat of the soul. But the DSM-5 provides an extremely thorough and comprehensive way of making diagnoses. The idea is to observe the characteristics and behaviors of people who appear to have a psychiatric disease such as depression, schizophrenia, or substance abuse and then compare their behavior to that of another person exhibiting similar symptoms to determine if they fit some of the same criteria.

Now, a crucial caveat with statistics—which are all-too often misleading, as anyone knows—is to understand the assumptions and methods under which they were collected, and put them in a proper context. For the DSM, statistics are gathered from individuals who have no other "regular" medical problems. Indeed, kidney or liver disease, or even simple infections, can cause build-up of substances in the body that can act on the brain, causing people to behave as if they are "crazy" or having other psychiatric problems. In general, it is usually not difficult for a good doctor to sort out strange behaviors due to most medical problems as opposed to "pure" psychiatric ones. (The exception to this, interestingly, is neurologic diseases. These diseases can present with very insidious, complex, and subtle behavior changes that can be most difficult to differentiate, sort out, or distinguish from psychiatric ones.)

The DSM had a most unlikely beginning, that of the 1840 United States Census. The 1840 census year was the first to include individuals in the category of "idiocy/insanity." In 1843, the American Statistical Association protested to the U.S. House of Representatives that the census data was gravely in error. In 1844, the Association of Medical Superintendents of American Institutions for the Insane, the ancestor of the current day American Psychiatric Association (APA), was born and published the first two issues of a journal *The American Journal of Insanity,* currently known as the *American Journal of Psychiatry.* The last article (American Journal of Insanity, 1844)[1] of the first issue contained statistics of the number of insane and idiotic patients in the U.S. by state, as well as an accounting of the lunatic asylums in the U.S.

In 1917, the APA developed a new guide for mental hospitals, called the *Statistical Manual for the Use of Institutions for the Insane.* It included 22 diagnoses, most of which remain as significant problems today: for example, manic depression, problems associated with alcohol and drug abuse, and psychiatric disease associated with medical conditions such as stroke, vitamin deficiency, and infections such as syphilis. In 1952, under the direction of Brigadier General and psychiatrist William Menninger, the APA brought forth the first edition of the DSM, the DSM-I. It was 130 pages long and listed 106 diagnoses. DSM-II came out in 1968; it was 134 pages and listed 182 diagnoses. These early editions of the DSM took a Freudian analytic approach to mental disease. Some doctors thought the criteria were diagnostically unreliable. In 1980, a greatly expanded and overhauled DSM-III was published. This edition of the DSM was spearheaded by, and to a great extent much of it was written by, psychiatrist Robert Spitzer. The DSM-III was 494 pages long and had 265 diagnostic categories! The DSM-III abandoned the Freudian approach as its framework, and instead applied the more systematic characterization of psychiatric diagnoses of 19th century German psychiatrist Emil Kraeplin. As well, the DSM-III began to base diagnoses on principles and findings from the developing field of neuroscience. The DSM-IV and DSM-5 relied on thousands of doctors and scientists studying and evaluating clinical and basic science evidence to revise the DSM-III. The DSM-5 (published in 2013) is 947 pages long and has nearly 300 diagnoses.

The current edition of the DSM emphasizes that, when making psychiatric diagnoses, it is important not only to consider disorders such as major depression, bipolar ("manic") depression, substance abuse, schizo-phrenia, and anxiety disorders, to name a few, but also severe personality disorders, as well as general medical and neurologic diseases that can pro-duce psychiatric symptoms (e.g., Alzheimer's dementia or delirium from severe infection or electrolyte imbalances). (Interestingly, in great litera-ture the author quite often will go to great extent and/or detail to exclude general medical problems.) We also must consider the life stressors that can exacerbate psychiatric disease, and also the severity—mild, moderate, severe, very severe—of psychiatric disease.

It's fascinating to observe that, despite how complicated we think the mind and its afflictions may be, there's really just a handful of ways that such disorders are currently categorized. Indeed, can there be only a small handful of common ways that the mind can fail psychiatrically? In this book, however, we can and will look at "patients presenting" themselves to readers in works of fiction. For fun and for the purposes of this book (as well as a way to explain the DSM-5), let's consider that we have a psy-chiatric "clinic" consisting of literary characters from any work of fiction. What I have found is that occasionally there is a character that some-times centuries or even millennia ahead of the formal medical/scientific description exhibits all the characteristics of one of the DSM-5 diagnoses. These are not just vague descriptions or something recognizable now as the DSM disease, but descriptions that in many cases are even better than the current ones in textbooks! Most other fictional characters I have found are either not diseased at all, or just in some range of normal. Of course, no one can read everything to collect a "clinic" consisting of absolutely all characters in all fiction ever written. But we can try. Curiously, and some-thing I find more than a bit spooky, the longest article (American Jour-nal of Insanity, 1844)[2] in that first issue of the *American Journal of Insanity* was a study of insanity in history, literature, and poetry! I don't find any examples given in this article that meet DSM criteria for insanity (schizo-phrenia) or any related diagnoses. In this book, we'll return to literature as a vehicle to understand the DSM but also as a means to understand and probe the diseases themselves.

1

The Case of Samson,
Son of Manoah

THE BIBLICAL STORY OF SAMSON (Judges 13–16), the legendary strongman, hero of the Israelites who bravely fought against the Philistines until he was tricked by the deceitful Philistine Delilah into revealing the secret of his great strength—his legendary locks of hair—is one well-known in several faiths and beyond. This tragic tale is also one of revenge and sacrifice: The evil Philistines torture Samson by gouging out his eyes and leave the source of his strength, his locks of hair, intact and force him to do manual labor. Yet Samson gets his vengeance by pulling down the foundation of a Philistine temple—crushing not only himself, but also the Philistines who were mocking him inside.

But upon closer scrutiny, not all is so clear—at least in the moral sense—in the Biblical story from all those millennia ago. Something more is going on here. Samson's actions are not always heroic and often are inexplicable in terms of the simple stuff of legend. It is with the help of modern medicine that we can peel away the sophisticated psychological profile subtly told by the unknown author, thousands of years ago, in this story about faith.

To begin at the beginning of the story, it's really curious that fully one-quarter of the Samson story is devoted to Samson's mother and Samson's difficult entry into the world. Unable to conceive a child, Samson's mother was in the fields when angels came to her and told her not to drink alcohol, and that only then she would have a child. After returning from the encounter in the fields with the angels, Samson's mother became pregnant.

But why was Samson's mother admonished so strongly not to drink alcohol? Difficulty in conception is a common theme in the Old Testament: In the book of Genesis, Abraham's wife, Sarah, Isaac's wife, Rebecca, and Rachel, one of Jacob's wives, all had trouble conceiving. But no angel ever pointed to laying off the wine as a key to getting pregnant.

That's just the first mystery of the Samson saga. Another curiosity is how alone he is—and how his fights with those villainous Philistines erupt time and time again. Samson is not a military leader like Moses or Joshua; he never leads troops in any pitched battles. Instead, he's just involved in street fights, pitting himself alone against large numbers of Philistines.

Many of Samson's actions—killing a group of men for their clothes to pay off a losing wager, frequenting brothels, perpetrating large-scale vandalism—are totally at odds with the simple, tragic tale popularly held of the Herculean, brave, and intrepid defender of the Israelite state. Obviously, it's at least a bit baffling that this Israelite hero is arrested by his own people. And it's almost always forgotten that Samson himself brings on his own destruction when he tells Delilah the all-important secret of his strength—even though she already tried to kill him three times.

Remarkably, Samson's quirks, baffling actions, and self-destruction fit into a modern profile of a mentally ill mind that has been "officially diagnosed" for less than 100 years. The psychiatric disease first formally described in the 20th Century is called antisocial personality disorder, or ASPD—and it completely explains Samson's actions, his motivations, his crimes, and, ultimately, his downfall. The Judges author was so far ahead of his time in "diagnosing" Samson, it's absolutely uncanny. In modern times, meeting three of seven very-specific criteria (as defined by the DSM-5) equals a diagnosis of ASPD—actions such as murder, robbery, arrests, reckless disregard of the safety of oneself or others (such as telling someone like Delilah the secret to taking away your strength after she has already tried to kill you three times!). Somehow, incredibly, the writer of the Samson story, working three thousand years ago, seemed to know all seven of these criteria; Samson clearly meets six of the seven—and the writer clearly, and knowingly, nods at the seventh and final criterion, as well (Altschuler et al., 2001).

ASPD

Curiously, there are now many quite good treatments for the most common psychiatric disorders, such as depression and schizophrenia, but few if any for the major personality disorders (such as borderline personality disorder, narcissistic personality disorder and ASPD). Indeed, there are currently no specifically approved drugs to treat ASPD. The only "treatment" often is incarceration. But interestingly enough, ASPD can sometimes "burn out" as affected individuals age.

Now, let us put Samson in his rightful place in this context. Remember when considering a psychiatric diagnosis, first we must rule out general medical problems that may contribute to, or influence, the psychiatric symptoms. Samson is portrayed as nothing but a healthy and vibrant young man with no significant medical problems.

TABLE 1.1 ⌁ **Diagnostic Criteria for Antisocial Personality Disorder**

A. There is a pervasive pattern of disregard for and violation of the rights of others occurring since age 15 years, as indicated by three (or more) of the following:

  1. Failure to conform to social norms with respect to lawful behaviors as indicated by repeatedly performing acts that are grounds for arrest

  2. Deceitfulness, as indicated by repeated lying, use of aliases, or conning others for personal profit or pleasure

  3. Impulsivity or failure to plan ahead

  4. Irritability and aggressiveness, as indicated by repeated physical fights or assaults

  5. Reckless disregard for safety of self or others

  6. Consistent irresponsibility, as indicated by repeated failure to sustain consistent work behavior or honor financial obligations

  7. Lack of remorse, as indicated by being indifferent to or rationalizing having hurt, mistreated, or stolen from another

B. The individual is at least age 18 years.

C. There is evidence of conduct disorder (see Table 1.2, below) with onset before age 15 years.

D. The occurrence of antisocial behavior is not exclusively during the course of schizophrenia or a manic episode.

(Reprinted with permission from the *Diagnostic and Statistical Manual of Mental Disorders, Fifth Edition,* © 2013. American Psychiatric Association.)

A modern patient needs to meet three of seven criteria (Table 1.1) to receive a diagnosis of ASPD. Since Samson is a fictional character, we are not able to examine him or run tests to absolutely convince ourselves that he does not have any other medical problems. So in this case, and in general, it's prudent not to make a diagnosis of a literary figure unless that figure not only meets, but greatly exceeds, the modern criteria necessary for diagnosis. This way, we can be pretty certain that the individual does not have some other disease affecting their behavior. For example, if the character exhibits six of the seven criteria, as opposed to three of the seven for the requirement of a diagnosing a current modern patient, it would appear that the writer has deliberately written things so as to fit the diagnosis. I actually think that historical cases are thus the best verification that the DSM-5 is representing real and natural phenomena, not just the product of too many modern committee meetings. The only way that the writer would seem to be able to possibly know the criteria is to have carefully observed a case or cases.

Samson, with his troubled history, meets six of the seven criteria for ASPD (Altschuler et al., 2001). But in a clever way the writer is also letting us know that he knows the seventh criterion, and toys with that, too.

Most of the criteria Samson meets more than once, and the author rein-forces this point again and again, just to make sure we get it. Also, criteria are often met in a clear way. For example, one criterion for ASPD is reck-less disregard of safety of self. Well, Samson took on 1000 men all by him-self in one encounter. Disregard of safety of self might be taking on two or three men at once. Reckless disregard of safety of self might be taking on ten men at once. Samson takes this to a hyperbolic extreme in taking on a thousand at once! The Judges tale shows, point by diagnostic point:

1. Failure to conform to social norms with respect to lawful behavior: The Philistines tried to arrest Samson after he burned the Philistine fields (15:5) and went to Gaza (16:1).

2. Deceitfulness, as indicated by repeated lying: Samson did not tell his parents that he had killed a lion. Furthermore, he proffered honey for his parents to eat, but did not tell them it had come from the carcass of a lion (14:9) and thus caused them to violate their dietary laws. Samson also demonstrated deceitfulness or cunning in using a riddle that it would be impossible for the interlocutors to answer (Judges 14:12–14).

3. Impulsivity: His burning of the Philistine fields (15:5).

4. Irritability and aggressiveness: This is indicated by his repeated involvement in physical fights, almost none of which are planned or organized beforehand. They're basically hotheaded brawls.

5. Reckless disregard for safety of self or others: Samson is reported to have taken on and killed 1000 Philistines single-handedly (15:15). To translate this mathematically: if one individual takes on one thousand, this one individual would have to believe in having a probability of greater than 99.93% of beating each opponent to even assume to have a 50% chance of surviving the fight. Similarly, telling Delilah the secret to his strength (16:17)—even after she had obviously attempted three times previously to get this secret—can also be considered reckless disregard for safety of self.

6. Lack of remorse: He gloated (15:16) after killing 1000 men.

7. The only criterion for ASPD that Samson does not meet is failure to meet one's financial obligations. However, the author of the story (with a wink and a nod) betrays knowledge of this criterion as well when he has Samson repay his lost bet only by killing 30 men, and using the stolen dead men's garments to pay up (Judges 14:19). So the author knows all seven criteria for ASPD and is clearly letting us know that he knows.

In addition to these adult criteria, to diagnose ASPD an individual must meet criteria when he was a youth. Unbelievably—and again, as if the writer had a 3,000-year advance copy of the DSM—the author lays them out as if he were a textbook example. Samson committed many of the actions listed in the criteria for conduct disorder (Table 1.2)—fire setting,

---

TABLE 1.2 ⚜ **Diagnostic Criteria for Conduct Disorder**

A. A repetitive and persistent pattern of behavior in which the basic rights of others or major age-appropriate societal norms or rules are violated, as manifested by the presence of three (or more) of the following criteria in the past twelve months, with at least one criterion present in the past six months.

Aggression to people and animals, or:

1. Often bullies, threatens, or intimidates others
2. Often initiates physical fights
3. Has used a weapon that can cause serious physical harm to others (e.g., a bat, brick, broken bottle, knife, gun)
4. Has been physically cruel to people
5. Has been physically cruel to animals
6. Has stolen while confronting a victim (e.g., mugging, purse snatching, extortion, armed robbery)
7. Has forced someone into sexual activity

Has committed some form of property destruction:

8. Has deliberately engaged in fire setting with the intention of causing serious damage
9. Has deliberately destroyed others' property (other than by setting fires)

Is guilty of deceitfulness or theft:

10. Has broken into someone else's house, building, or car
11. Often lies to obtain goods or favors or to avoid obligations (i.e., "cons" others)
12. Has stolen items of nontrivial value without confronting a victim (e.g., shoplifting, but without breaking and entering; forgery)

Is somehow in serious violations of established rules:

13. Often stays out at night despite parental prohibitions, beginning before age 13 years
14. Has run away from home overnight at least twice while living in parental or parental surrogate home (or once without returning for a lengthy period)
15. Is often truant from school, beginning before age 13 years

B. The disturbance in behavior causes clinically significant impairment in social, academic, or occupational functioning.

(Reprinted with permission from the *Diagnostic and Statistical Manual of Mental Disorders, Fifth Edition*, © 2013. American Psychiatric Association.)

cruelty to small animals (15:5), bullying, initiating physical fights, using a weapon (like the donkey's jawbone) (15:15), and stealing from a victim (14:19). If the preliminary conduct disorder did not start when Samson was younger than 15 years, he was still quite young (14:1–6).

DSM diagnoses require not only to meet various criteria—the **inclusion criteria**—but also to *not* have other criteria—the **exclusion criteria**. Samson shows no evidence of schizophrenia. Some of his behaviors (e.g., not telling his parents that the honey had been taken from a carcass) were performed during a clearly non-manic state.

Now, besides excluding general medical conditions and other psychiatric disease, and meeting all inclusion and exclusion criteria for ASPD, a further criterion one might want Samson to meet is that somehow his behavior wasn't simply some kind of normal response to a difficult experience or circumstance. Indeed, one might argue that the era of the Judges was a violent one, a time when people went around lying, stealing, and committing arson and murder. A relativistic and modern reading of the text might suggest that we cannot necessarily impose our definition of capital murder on Samson's murder of 30 men for their clothes.

But the author seems aware of this possible objection and shows that Samson's conduct is clearly unacceptable even in his own time—as 3000 Israelites (Samson's own people) capture him and deliver him to the Philistines (15:12). Furthermore, unlike Moses, Joshua, Saul, or David, Samson never led any great armies in battles or even fought in a battle on behalf of his people. Instead, he simply instigated fights, and killed, for no reason.

Samson's ASPD explains some other mysteries about the story. To begin with, the first out of four chapters on Samson tells the story of how Samson's mother got pregnant: her experience meeting someone in a field who told her not to drink alcohol while pregnant. This is odd because while difficulty conceiving is a common theme in the Old Testament (e.g., Sarah wife of Abraham, Rebecca wife of Isaac, and Rachel one of Jacob's wives) no one had to tell these women not to drink alcohol when they were pregnant. In fact, there are circumstances quite to the contrary; when Hannah, the mother of Samuel, was praying at the Temple altar while having trouble conceiving, Temple elders who overheard her prayers actually asked her if she was drunk—the prayers having apparently been so mournful— but Hannah responded that of course she did not drink.

It appears Samson's mother *needed* to be told not to drink because she did drink. The author of the Samson story somehow knew and is relating that ASPD has a genetic component, and that indeed it tends to manifest in women as substance abuse and promiscuity, and in men as violence.

Finally, there is Samson's death and its unusual manner. The natural history of ASPD is that if the disease does not burn itself out with the sufferer becoming less antisocial (more social) over time, then the individual with ASPD often times winds up incarcerated or dead in a violent way, likely from homicide or suicide. The manner in which Samson died is really a suicide. In religious teachings it is often couched as a heroic act against the hated Philistines. But surely almost all the individuals in the Philistine temple crushed alongside Samson were innocent. So by shoving the pillars and bringing down the temple Samson tallied up one final mass murder. This act was impulsive, aggressive, and with reckless disregard for the safety of himself and others, and thus at once meets and emphasizes multiple ASPD criteria, all in one final push.

The case of Samson illustrates that ASPD itself is an old disease. Today, ASPD is thought to be at the end of a final common pathway resulting from a combination of genetic and environmental factors such as early brain damage from trauma or other causes. Thus, as such factors have been around from time immemorial, we would expect ASPD to be an old disease. It's amazing and satisfying to find confirmation of this expectation, hidden in plain sight in The Holy Bible.

2

Using the DSM-5
The Oldest Case of Schizophrenia Found in a Story by Nicolai Gogol

AS WE JUST LEARNED IN CHAPTER 1, the "case" of Samson shows us that ASPD is a disorder that's almost as old as history itself, with presumably genetics, trauma, and other environmental factors contributing and combining to cause brain damage resulting in the disorder. One might hazard a guess that schizophrenia—now so common, affecting about one percent of the population—might also be documented over the millennia. However, no descriptions of a disease resembling schizophrenia can be found before 1800 (Haslam, 1798; Pinel, 1801).

What changed in the modern world? After 1800, descriptions of schizophrenia began to appear, and then grow in number (Hare, 1988; Haslam, 1809; Pinel, 1809). For example, casebooks from both England and the European continent start to describe patients at "mental" asylums who might have schizophrenia, but only beginning with the literature published after 1800 (Haslam, 1798, 1809; Hare, 1988; Pinel, 1801, 1809). Truly, schizophrenia is a detailed condition that needs to be scientifically parsed out from other common conditions and diseases, such as substance abuse and mania, which often present the same symptoms as schizophrenia. Interestingly, the remarkable short story *Diary of a Madman* by the great Ukranian/Russian litterateur, Nicolai Gogol (1809–1852) has the earliest, clearest, and—as we will see time and again from great writers—the most complete description of schizophrenia (Altschuler, 2001).

In lay terms we tend to refer to people with schizophrenia as being "crazy." But this is a narrow definition of this kind of crazy. The DSM-5 criteria for schizophrenia are given in Table 2.1. When trying to diagnose schizophrenia today or study its antiquity, it is essential to rule out other diseases and conditions. Substance misuse or withdrawal could lead to "crazy" speech by an individual. Heavy metal poisoning—either deliberate or inadvertent from metals in the food or water chain—could also

TABLE 2.1 Diagnostic Criteria for Schizophrenia

A. **Characteristic symptoms**: Two (or more) of the following, including at least one of the first three, each present for a significant portion of time during a 1-month period (or less if successfully treated):

1. Delusions

2. Hallucinations

3. Disorganized speech (e.g., frequent derailment or incoherence)

4. Grossly disorganized or catatonic behavior

5. Negative symptoms (i.e., affective flattening, alogia, or avolition)

B. **Social/occupational dysfunction**: For a significant portion of the time since the onset of the disturbance, one or more major areas of functioning such as work, interpersonal relations, or self-care are markedly below the level achieved prior to the onset (or when the onset is in childhood or adolescence, failure to achieve expected level of interpersonal, academic, or occupational achievement).

C. **Duration**: Continuous signs of the disturbance persist for at least 6 months. This 6-month period must include at least 1 month of symptoms (or less if successfully treated) that meet Criterion A (i.e., active-phase symptoms) and may include periods of prodromal or residual symptoms. During these prodromal or residual periods, the signs of the disturbance may be manifested by only negative symptoms or two or more symptoms listed in Criterion A present in an attenuated form (e.g., odd beliefs, unusual perceptual experiences).

D. **Schizoaffective and Mood Disorder exclusion**: Schizoaffective disorder and mood disorder with psychotic features have been ruled out because either: 1. no major depressive, manic, or mixed episodes have occurred concurrently with the active-phase symptoms; or 2. if mood episodes have occurred during active-phase symptoms, their total duration has been brief relative to the duration of the active and residual periods.

E. **Substance/general medical condition exclusion**: The disturbance is not due to the direct physiological effects of a substance (e.g., a drug of abuse, a medication) or a general medical condition.

F. **Relationship to a Pervasive Developmental Disorder**: If there is a history of autistic disorder or another pervasive developmental disorder, the additional diagnosis of schizophrenia is made only if prominent delusions or hallucinations are also present for at least a month (or less if successfully treated).

(Reprinted with permission from the *Diagnostic and Statistical Manual of Mental Disorders, Fifth Edition,* © 2013. American Psychiatric Association.)

lead to these symptoms; and so could vitamin deficiencies (deficiencies of pellagra, niacin, Vitamin B3, for example). People who are just manic (or in the manic phase of bipolar disease) can also "talk crazy."

Along with the exclusion criteria necessary to diagnose schizophrenia, we need to look at the inclusion criteria, as well. The first four characteristic symptoms (Table 2.1, criteria A) are known as **positive symptoms** of schizophrenia (i.e., "excessive" speech or actions made by an individual with schizophrenia). Gogol, writing from 19th century Czarist Russia, seems to know all of these and also the exclusion criteria a century before they were described as being part of the disease. But people with schizophrenia can also exhibit the **negative symptoms** listed in Table 2.1 (number 5 in criteria A). In these cases individuals with schizophrenia exhibit these kinds of speech or actions much *less* than normal individuals. While Gogol knows all of the positive symptoms of schizophrenia, he either does not know (or simply does not mention) the negative symptoms. The modern recognition of the negative symptoms of schizophrenia may reflect more difficulty in appreciating them on the part of clinicians, or that negative symptoms represent a disease variant with its own etiology and history.

But the Ukranian/Russian writer was certainly an amazingly acute observer of what is now a relatively common diagnosis in modern medicine. Gogol was born in the Ukraine in 1809 (Fanger, 1979). He moved to St. Petersburg in 1829 where he got a job through a friend at a government ministry. From 1834 to 1842 he published five tales about his native Ukraine, including *Diary of a Madman* (1834), *The Nose* (1836), and *The Overcoat* (1842). During this time period he wrote many other stories, essays, and plays. In 1842 he published part one of his magnum opus, the novel *Dead Souls*. Gogol spent much of his last years outside of Russia. In 1848 he made a pilgrimage to Jerusalem; apparently he had an increasing interest in religion in the ensuing years. He completed part two of *Dead Souls* in 1852, but then burnt the manuscript shortly thereafter and died a few weeks after that, perhaps from self-starvation. Gogol is considered one of the foundational figures of Russian literature. Indeed, Dostoevsky reportedly commented, "We all come out from Gogol's *Overcoat*."

Diary of a Madman is one of Gogol's masterly artistic statements. The protagonist, Poprishchin, is a forty-something Ukrainian civil servant, and the story takes the form of his diary entries of his descent into insanity. The first entry is for October 3rd (year 1). (Gogol's story does not list years, but it's helpful to try and enumerate them while cataloguing the progression of Poprishchin's condition). This October day starts poorly for Poprishchin, who sleeps too long and shows up late for work. Strangely, Poprishchin notes in his diary that later that day he thinks he hears two dogs talking to each other in Russian. He further notes: "It can't be true, I must be drunk. But I hardly ever drink." Things continue to get worse quickly for Poprishchin; he has increasing trouble at work, and on November 13th (year 1) he notes that he reads letters from the dogs to each other.

Shortly thereafter, (December 5th, year 1) Poprishchin notes in his diary that he read in the newspaper about the dispute of the succession of King Ferdinand VII of Spain (1833). Then on "April 43rd, 2000" (perhaps April of year 2?) Poprishchin makes a great leap, writing: "Today is a day of great triumph. There is a king of Spain. He has been found at last. That king is me. I only discovered this today." The very next entry in the diary is dated "86th Martober, between day and night" (October of year 2?). Poprishchin goes to work after a three-week absence and he behaves offensively to his boss and coworkers. Later, in an entry prefaced "No date," Poprishchin writes that he had been in a large crowd but "did not reveal [his] identity [as King Ferdinand VIII]." The date of the last entry of the diary is **"Da 34 te Mth eary ɟǝqɯnɐɹʎ 349"** (February of year 3?). Poprishchin writes that people are pouring cold water over his head; his head is spinning; the sky whirls.

Thus, starting possibly in April of the second year of his madness, Poprishchin has the persistent delusion that he is King of Spain. This delusion continues for the rest of the story, a period lasting at least three weeks—the time that he did not go to work—but probably lasting months or even longer. His condition progressively worsens, and throughout this time he demonstrates disorganized behavior and occupational dysfunction by not going to work and acting bizarrely when he does. But even before the start of the delusion that he is the King of Spain (not coincidentally dated with a diary entry with a bizarre date "April 43, 2000"), Poprishchin experiences a "prodromal" period, which includes the hallucinations that dogs are speaking to each other in a human language and the hallucination or delusion that the dogs are even writing letters to each other. The text of the diary shows that Poprishchin's speech and language is becoming increasingly disordered, the date of the final entry of the diary being just one example of this.

Along with all the inclusion criteria for schizophrenia (positive symptoms), Poprishchin also demonstrates a symptom of schizophrenia called **ideas of reference** (a symptom Gogol is aware of and has the earliest vivid description of). In modern times these ideas of reference commonly manifest themselves as the notion that a television newscaster or other television personality is speaking directly to the schizophrenic patient. In Gogol's story, ideas of reference manifest when Poprishchin reads about the trouble with the succession of the King of Spain, and takes the problem personally, which is absurd and completely inappropriate because he is not even a citizen of Spain.

There is no evidence that Poprishchin has a pervasive developmental disorder, major depression, or a general medical condition. He does not demonstrate any of the typical behavioral signs of mania such as going without sleep, hypersexuality, or profligate spending. Mania can produce delusions such as that one is a King. However, if Poprishchin were manic, we might expect such a delusion to manifest itself differently. Indeed, in the diary entry dated "No date," Poprishchin says that he was in a crowd but did not point out to anyone that they were in the presence of a king. A manic patient would perhaps take such an opportunity to make a grand pronouncement of their importance. Also, there is no evidence of substance misuse or dependence by Poprishchin, and alcoholism is explicitly ruled out when he writes from the outset: "But I hardly ever drink." This exclusion is important as alcohol misuse or dependence is not uncommon in Gogol's writings. And while Poprishchin is rather old (in his 40s) for a first onset of schizophrenia, it's not unheard of today.

Diary of a Madman is one of the oldest and certainly most complete early description of schizophrenia. With the exception of the omission of the negative symptoms, this story is a total sketch of schizophrenia, the same way that Samson's tale seems an outline of ASPD. And, like the Samson story, it is as if Gogol wrote this sketch using the DSM criteria for schizophrenia, yet the DSM lay a century in the future. The story certainly suggests strongly that there must have been a real case or cases in the Ukraine or Russia that Gogol observed. However, the influence of literary characters such as Kapellemeister Kreisler, a creation of German writer E. T. A. Hoffmann (1776–1822) cannot be ruled out. Indeed, Gogol's original title was *The Diary of a Mad Musician* (Fanger, 1979 p. 115), itself a nod to Hoffmann who, besides being a writer, was a composer and music critic. Hoffmann's works are extensive and complex, and contain many curious characters in their own right. But in all of them there are no cases of schizophrenia, and certainly no descriptions written with the pure clarity and unequivocal manner of Gogol's case. Gogol may have been inspired by reports in newspapers such as *The Northern Bee* (which Gogol actually ridicules and satirizes to great effect in *Diary of a Madman*), about inmates at insane asylums (Fanger, 1979). Further study of these reports and the works of Hoffmann for cases of schizophrenia might be warranted, however. Gogol's apparent case of schizophrenia in the Ukraine or Russia (or even Germany) observed no later than 1834—when thought about in conjunction with other cases in England and France in 1809 (Hare, 1988; Haslam, 1809; Pinel, 1809)— reveal that schizophrenia was already common in Europe by early in the 19th century, making it increasingly unlikely, though not impossible, that schizophrenia was a new fascinating phenomenon—and was undocumented before 1800.

If schizophrenia is an old disease, then why are there so few early reports? There are at least four possible explanations:

1. The increase in the reported number of cases of schizophrenia may be an artifact of the tremendous increase in the number of physicians and medical researchers in the past 200 years.

2. Modern descriptions of schizophrenia, starting with that by German psychiatrist Emil Kraepelin in 1898 (Kohl, 1999), have greatly facilitated the recognition of schizophrenia by clinicians, thus possibly accounting for the tremendous increase in cases. That is, the number of cases of schizophrenia was always high but just

weren't recognized, appreciated, or properly classified by physicians.

3. A DSM diagnosis of schizophrenia requires diminished social functioning, and most people with schizophrenia in the past would have been unable to write or ensure dissemination of information about their condition. Furthermore, given the typical downtrodden plight of people with chronic (untreated) schizophrenia, those with the disease may not have been an enticing topic for description by non-patient authors.

4. Finally, there may indeed be some aetiological agent, new or absent, since 1800 responsible for the great increase in the number of cases, but that agent remains unknown.

Further checking of medical, literary, and other written sources may yield additional old cases of schizophrenia. Increased confidence that schizophrenia is an old disease, or not, may help in forming hypotheses and guiding research to find better methods to treat or prevent this common and highly morbid disease[1].

3

A Hoarding Old Man and a Disembodied Nose
Other Diagnoses in Gogol

Hoarding Disorder in *Dead Souls*

MOST INTERESTINGLY AND CURIOUSLY, schizophrenia is not the only pioneering, complete DSM diagnosis in Gogol's works. Hoarding disorder is listed as a new diagnosis in DSM-5 with presumed unique neurobiological correlates, and not just as a symptom of obsessive-compulsive personality disorder as it was in DSM-IV. However, this would not be news to Gogol who wrote about this disorder in his masterpiece *Dead Souls* (1842).

In Part One of Gogol's *Dead Souls* (1842), the protagonist Chichikov is a con man and former bureaucrat who tours around the countryside looking for minor landowners from whom to buy dead peasant souls as part of a money-making tax evasion scheme. (Chichikov plans to buy the deceased souls from landowners on the cheap, and then, in an arbitrage based on the relative infrequency of the census, claim a tax break for himself on the souls.) In Chapter 6, the most curious individual Chichikov meets is Plyushkin, who, even from the short quotes below, is clearly seen to have hoarding disorder (Hogarth, 1916; Cybulska, 1998).

> *"Entering a large, dark hall which reeked like a tomb, he passed into an equally dark parlor that was lighted only by such rays as contrived to filter through a crack under the door. When Chichikov opened the door in question, the spectacle of the untidiness within struck him almost with amazement. It would seem that the floor was never washed, and that the room was used as a receptacle for every conceivable kind of furniture. On a table stood a ragged chair, with, beside it, a clock minus a pendulum and covered all over with cobwebs. Against a wall leant a cupboard, full of old silver, glassware, and china. On a writing*

table, inlaid with mother-of-pearl which, in places, had broken away and left behind it a number of yellow grooves (stuffed with putty), lay a pile of finely written manuscript, an overturned marble press (turning green), an ancient book in a leather cover with red edges, a lemon dried and shrunken to the dimensions of a hazelnut, the broken arm of a chair, a tumbler containing the dregs of some liquid and three flies (the whole covered over with a sheet of notepaper), a pile of rags, two ink-encrusted pens, and a yellow toothpick with which the master of the house had picked his teeth (apparently) at least before the coming of the French to Moscow. As for the walls, they were hung with a medley of pictures. Among the latter was a long engraving of a battle scene, wherein soldiers in three-cornered hats were brandishing huge drums and slender lances. It lacked a glass, and was set in a frame ornamented with bronze fretwork and bronze corner rings. Beside it hung a huge, grimy oil painting representative of some flowers and fruit, half a watermelon, a boar's head, and the pendent form of a dead wild duck. Attached to the ceiling there was a chandelier in a holland covering—the covering so dusty as closely to resemble a huge cocoon enclosing a caterpillar. Lastly, in one corner of the room lay a pile of articles which had evidently been adjudged unworthy of a place on the table. Yet what the pile consisted of it would have been difficult to say, seeing that the dust on the same was so thick that any hand which touched it would have at once resembled a glove. Prominently protruding from the pile was the shaft of a wooden spade and the antiquated sole of a shoe. Never would one have supposed that a living creature had tenanted the room, were it not that the presence of such a creature was betrayed by the spectacle of an old nightcap resting on the table."

"… the most noticeable feature about the man was his clothes. In no way could it have been guessed of what his coat was made, for both its sleeves and its skirts were so ragged and filthy as to defy description, while instead of two posterior tails, there dangled four of those appendages, with, projecting from them, a torn newspaper. Also, around his neck there was wrapped something which might have been a stocking, a garter, or a stomacher, but was certainly not a tie. In short, had Chichikov chanced to encounter him at a church door, he would have bestowed upon him a copper or two (for, to do our hero justice, he had a sympathetic heart and never refrained from presenting a beggar with alms), but in the present case there was standing before him, not a mendicant, but a landowner—and a landowner possessed of fully a thousand serfs, the superior of all his neighbours in wealth of flour and grain, and the owner of storehouses, and so forth, that were crammed with homespun cloth and linen,

tanned and undressed sheepskins, dried fish, and every conceivable
species of produce. Nevertheless, such a phenomenon is rare in Russia,
where the tendency is rather to prodigality than to parsimony."

Moreover, Plyushkin wanders the streets of his village on a daily basis looking, amongst other places, under bridges and in puddles to pick up any old shoe sole, rag, iron nail or pottery shard to put in the pile of junk in the moldy house. Plyushkin has excessive acquisitiveness and little, if any, insight into his disorder.

Gogol implicitly suggests knowledge far beyond just the signs of hoarding disorder. He describes the trajectory by which Plyushkin ended up in the state in which Chichikov met him: Plyushkin was a thrifty proprietor. Then his wife died. His older daughter ran off with an army officer. His son, having been schooled for the civil service, enlisted in a regiment. His younger daughter died. The result was Plyushkin, a man who spiraled into miserliness, and eventually exhibited the characteristics of hoarding disorder. It will be interesting to see if Plyushkin's trajectory will be the same as the modern one for patients diagnosed with this "new" disorder. The DSM-5 criteria for Hoarding Disorder are listed in Table 3.1 on page 22.

Dissociative Amnesia and *The Nose*

Part One of Gogol's *The Nose* (1836) opens on March 25th with the barber Ivan Yakovlevich finding a nose in his morning bread. Yakovlevich recognizes the nose as belonging to his customer Collegiate Assessor Kovalyov ("Major Kovalyov"). Yakovlevich's wife condemns Yakovlevich as a drunk; the narrator confirms this. Yakovlevich tries to dispose of the nose so he doesn't get in trouble with the law, but is thwarted in attempts to do so, finally being questioned by a policeman on a bridge over the Neva River as to his reason for being there.

Part Two opens with Major Kovalyov awakening and looking in a mirror to evaluate a pimple on his nose that had started to break out the day before. Kovalyov is shocked to find that instead of a pimple, he has no nose at all! Kovalyov confirms the absence by feeling for his nose and not finding it. Lamenting his absence of a nose, Kovalyov hits the streets and actually finds the nose sitting next to him—as a person—at Kazan Cathedral. The nose refuses to go back onto Kovalyov's face, so Kovalyov goes to the police. The police chief is not in, so he goes to a newspaper office to place an ad regarding the missing facial part but is refused. Kovalyov finds the police commissioner at his house but is told it's not a time for investigations.

Kovalyov goes home and pines for the loss of his nose. He feels like he must be dreaming or that he is drunk. To test this theory Kovalyov pinches himself strongly, and cries out from pain, thus convincing him-

TABLE 3.1 Diagnostic Criteria for Hoarding Disorder

A. Persistent difficulty discarding or parting with possessions, regardless of their actual value.

B. This difficulty is due to a perceived need to save the items and to distress associated with discarding them.

C. The difficulty discarding possessions results in the accumulation of possessions that congest and clutter active living areas and substantially compromises their intended use. If living areas are uncluttered, it is only because of the interventions of third parties (e.g., family members, cleaners, authorities).

D. The hoarding causes clinically significant distress or impairment in social, occupational, or other important areas of functioning (including maintaining a safe environment for self and others).

E. The hoarding is not attributable to another medical condition (e.g., brain injury, cerebrovascular disease, Prader-Willi syndrome).

F. The hoarding is not better explained by the symptoms of another mental disorder (e.g., obsessions in obsessive-compulsive disorder, decreased energy in major depressive disorder, delusions in schizophrenia or another psychotic disorder, cognitive deficits in major neurocognitive disorder, restricted interests in autism spectrum disorder).

Specify if:

With excessive acquisition: If difficulty discarding possessions is accompanied by excessive acquisition of items that are not needed or for which there is no available space.

Specify if:

With good or fair insight: The individual recognizes that hoarding-related beliefs and behaviors (pertaining to difficulty discarding items, clutter, or excessive acquisition) are problematic.

With poor insight: The individual is mostly convinced that hoarding-related beliefs and behaviors (pertaining to difficulty discarding items, clutter, or excessive acquisition) are not problematic despite evidence to the contrary.

With absent insight/delusional beliefs: The individual is completely convinced that hoarding-related beliefs and behaviors (pertaining to difficulty discarding items, clutter, or excessive acquisition) are not problematic despite evidence to the contrary.

self that he is not drunk. Soon after, a policeman arrives at Kovalyov's house with his nose and blames the barber Yakovlevich—who the policeman criticizes as being a drunkard and a thief. After the policeman leaves, Kovalyov calls a doctor to reattach his nose, but the doctor refuses to do so saying it is better to leave his face the way it is.

Part Three of the story takes place on April 7th. Kovalyov wakes up and feels his nose in its rightful place on his face, which he confirms by looking in the mirror. Then Kovalyov has an uneventful shave from Yakovlevich. The narrator attributes the events of the story to the strange supernatural. But, as we can see from Table 3.2, Kovalyov meets all the DSM-5 criteria for an episode of dissociative amnesia with dissociative fugue. In particular, a key moment is when Kovalyov confirms he is not drunk—the dissociative fugue not being attributable to alcohol misuse. Recall in *Diary of a Madman* when Poprischin explicitly states he is not drunk when he hears dogs speaking to each other in Russian, thereby excluding alcohol misuse as a cause of the hallucinations. The absence of drinking in Kovalyov stands out further in the story as both Yakovlevich's wife and a police say that he is a drunk!

With these early, complete diagnoses, Gogol ranks as one of the greatest descriptive, diagnostic psychiatrists of all time. How Gogol came upon his psychiatric interest, observations, and knowledge is just one of the many mysteries of the life of this immortal writer. There are other diagnoses in Gogol. For example, one wonders if Gogol did not find (or write about) himself in the depression of Andrey Ivanovich Tentetninkov in Part Two of *Dead Souls* (Maguirre, 2004). We'll never know.

TABLE 3.2 🠪 Diagnostic Criteria for Dissociative Amnesia
A. An inability to recall important autobiographical information, usually of a traumatic or stressful nature, that is inconsistent with ordinary forgetting. **Note:** Dissociative amnesia most often consists of localized or selective amnesia for a specific event or events; or generalized amnesia for identity and life history.
B. The symptoms cause clinically significant distress or impairment in social, occupational, or other important areas of functioning.
C. The disturbance is not attributable to the physiological effects of a substance (e.g., alcohol or other drug of abuse, a medication) or a neurological or other medical condition (e.g., partial complex seizures, transient global amnesia, sequelae of a closed head injury/traumatic brain injury, other neurological condition).
D. The disturbance is not better explained by dissociative identity disorder, posttraumatic stress disorder, acute stress disorder, somatic symptom disorder, or major or mild neurocognitive disorder.
Specify if: **With dissociative fugue:** Apparently purposeful travel or bewildered wandering that is associated with amnesia for identity or for other important autobiographical information.

(Reprinted with permission from the *Diagnostic and Statistical Manual of Mental Disorders, Fifth Edition,* © 2013. American Psychiatric Association.)

4

The Case of Dr. Henry Jekyll, M.D., D.C.L., LL.D., FRS, Ph.D[1]

IN THE WINTER OF 1885 money was tight. A Scottish writer is desperate to support his family. A shilling Christmas stocking stuffer could turn life's tide. A new potion, that's the secret, our writer perhaps thinks.

This writer of course, was Robert Louis Stevenson, now best known as the author of the immortal *Strange Case of Dr. Jekyll and Mr. Hyde*. In his most famous story was the author ministering to a substance abuse problem of his own, now eponymously mistaken for a tale about a split personality?

Stevenson's character Dr. Jekyll has all the harrowing hallmarks of an addict. He shows ten of the eleven designated modern criteria for Substance Abuse Disorder. In fact, if read carefully (Altschuler and Wright, 2000), the novella is an unacknowledged primer—and indeed a most helpful and useful one—on substance abuse for patients, physicians, and families.

Traditionally readers diagnose poor Dr. Jekyll with dual or multiple personality disorder. In common usage, and even in scientific literature (Ezekowitz, 1998), the names "Jekyll" and "Hyde" have become synonymous with a "split" personality. However, given the extreme rarity of new onset multiple personality disorder in an adult male (Hocke and Schmidtke, 1998), and compared with the high frequency of substance dependence diagnoses in adult males, as well as the ubiquitous association of Hyde with Jekyll's ingestion of his homemade potion, and the clues Stevenson etches in the tale, a strong argument could be made that Jekyll's disordered personality and suffering can be explained by substance use disorder (Altschuler and Wright, 2000). Jekyll's profession seems not a coincidence: Substance use disorders are overrepresented in physicians. (The typical demographic for multiple personality disorder is young women who have suffered abuse.)

The DSM-5 requires that two of eleven criteria (Table 4.1) be met in a 1-year period for a diagnosis of Substance Use Disorder. Jekyll meets nine! He increasingly starts to use larger quantities of the substance,

TABLE 4.1 Diagnostic Criteria for Other (or Unknown) Substance Use Disorder

A. A problematic pattern of use of an intoxicating substance not able to be classified within the alcohol; caffeine; cannabis; hallucinogen (phencyclidine and others); inhalant; opioid; sedative, hypnotic, or anxiolytic; stimulant; or tobacco categories and leading to clinically significant impairment or distress, as manifested by at least two of the following, occurring within a 12-month period:

1. The substance is often taken in larger amounts or over a longer period than was intended.

2. There is a persistent desire or unsuccessful efforts to cut down or control use of the substance.

3. A great deal of time is spent in activities necessary to obtain the substance, use the substance, or recover from its effects.

4. Craving, or a strong desire or urge to use the substance.

5. Recurrent use of the substance resulting in a failure to fulfill major role obligations at work, school, or home.

6. Continued use of the substance despite having persistent or recurrent social or interpersonal problems caused or exacerbated by the effects of its use.

7. Important social, occupational, or recreational activities are given up or reduced because of use of the substance.

8. Recurrent use of the substance in situations in which it is physically hazardous.

9. Use of the substance is continued despite knowledge of having a persistent or recurrent physical or psychological problem that is likely to have been caused or exacerbated by the substance.

10. Tolerance, as defined by either of the following:

    a. A need for markedly increased amounts of the substance to achieve intoxication or desired effect.

    b. A markedly diminished effect with continued use of the same amount of the substance.

11. Withdrawal, as manifested by either of the following:

    a. The characteristic withdrawal syndrome for other (or unknown) substance.

    b. The substance (or a closely related substance) is taken to relieve or avoid withdrawal symptoms.

(Reprinted with permission from the *Diagnostic and Statistical Manual of Mental Disorders, Fifth Edition*, © 2013. American Psychiatric Association.)

eventually doubling or tripling the amount (Stevenson, 1886, page 90), and Jekyll himself notes that he is risking death by using more (see Criteria 1, 4, 9, and 10). Despite his attempt to stop taking the potion (for two months Jekyll abstains from his potion), he cannot hold out any longer, and gives in to his compulsion (pages 91–92) (see Criteria 2, 4). Jekyll notes that it takes increasingly long for Hyde's onset to wear off and leave Jekyll intact (see Criterion 3). His affliction leads Dr. Jekyll to become withdrawn and lose his profession, household, friends (page 41), and eventually his life to the substance (see Criteria 5, 6, 7). Eventually Dr. Jekyll experiences withdrawal and states, "I swear to God I will never set eyes on him [Hyde] again. I bind my honour to you that I am done with him [Hyde] in this world" (page 34). This is an empty promise that might ring familiar to anyone who's seen a friend or family member struggle with addiction.

What Was Dr. Jekyll's Substance?

While alcohol is and was the most common drug of abuse, and Stevenson himself was known to have used alcohol, for a number of reasons it cannot be Jekyll's drug of choice. First, Jekyll twice mentions alcohol by way of comparison to his potion (pages 82, 92), with the implication that his potion is more than mere ethanol. Also, the main symptom associated with taking the potion—the vivid perception that Hyde is smaller than Jekyll—does not seem consistent with alcohol dependence (Elwin, 1950; Pope-Hennessy, 1994). Other drugs that Stevenson was known to have used are hashish and opium (Elwin, 1950; Pope-Hennessy, 1994) but neither of these drugs should cause Hyde to appear to be smaller than Jekyll. As well, the often energetic activity of Hyde, including murder, would not be consistent with opium dependence.

Cocaine was available when *Dr. Jekyll and Mr. Hyde* was written, but, if anything, cocaine might make Hyde feel larger than Jekyll, not smaller.[2] Hallucinogenic drugs can cause a change in body image perception. Although LSD would not be synthesized until the 1900s, Stevenson might have tried naturally occurring hallucinogens such as mushrooms. Or maybe Stevenson happened upon a hallucinogen in the course of attempting to treat his tuberculosis. To leave room for readers' imaginations—the wonderful ambiguity of great art—I believe Stevenson ultimately left the identity of the drug somewhat vague. Further, decades *before* the appearance of the DSM's specific criteria for alcohol and drug use disorder, Stevenson extends and universalizes, extends and acknowledges, that even if the drug is unknown or unspecified one can still be dependent on it![3]

5

Melville's Bartleby
Why the Scrivener Preferred Not

EARLY IN HIGH SCHOOL WE READ *Bartleby the Scrivener* (1853) by the great, and also greatly troubled, American author Herman Melville (1819–1891). The story—about an individual named Bartleby who had just started working as a scrivener, or copyist, at a Wall Street firm—is dark and somewhat complex. Fall and winter were also dark the year I read the book, as was our school building—a 20th century structure with only a few years of use left. So, when I would sometimes look out the windows and out into passageways, Melville's 19th century depictions didn't seem too far removed. Thus, we were buoyed when the teacher said she was going to show us a movie of the story.

If you want, this is a point to read the story yourself and try to formulate your own diagnosis for Bartleby, or else read on and see how I came upon it.

The movie was dark, like the story, but easier to understand. It was interesting to watch Bartleby, who, for his first three days at his new firm, performed extraordinarily well doing more than a standard scrivener's amount of work. But then, on his fourth day, when asked to do various tasks Bartleby would often respond, "I prefer not to." Eventually, Bartleby would not do any assignments, always saying "I prefer not to." This line of Bartleby's evoked mirth and laughter from my classmates. But the film became much more difficult to watch by its end. Bartleby started living at the firm's office and appeared to stop eating. Eventually the attorney who owned Bartleby's firm moved the firm to a new building and went on vacation for a few days. When he came back, he found out that Bartleby was in jail for being a vagrant. The attorney went to visit Bartleby in jail. Bartleby said to the attorney, "I know you…and I want nothing to say to you…I know where I am."

After the movie was over someone in the class, or maybe it was the teacher, said that Bartleby was "catatonic," which gave us all a good laugh. Now, at that time in New York there were a lot of deinstitutionalized mentally ill patients—many of whom were suffering from schizophrenia—often living homeless on the streets, and we saw them frequently. Many of these patients had a home on their favorite corner or favorite car on certain subway routes, and they could reliably be found day after day shouting loudly their own individualized comments or delusional rants. But they also had periods when they would stand motionless or in bizarre postures. By definition, *catatonia* refers to alteration in limb movements, typically manifesting as extreme rigidity or inflexibility of limbs, but colloquially my classmates and I used the phrase "catatonic schizophrenia." (Read more about schizophrenia, the DSM-5 criteria, and Gogol's *Diary of a Madman* in Chapter 2.)

The story is definitely provocative, and we talked about it for some days after watching the movie. Something was clearly wrong with Bartleby—it seemed genuine and not just some "fictional" creation—but he didn't seem exactly like the people with schizophrenia we were familiar with. Interestingly, we didn't focus on the medical in the story, even though there is plenty of disease to go around: The other two scriveners at the firm, Turkey and Nippers, can only work effectively half of each day—Turkey in the mornings and Nippers in the afternoons—due to alcoholism and severe chronic indigestion and poor circulation in the arms, respectively.

Thus, I was most fascinated and pleased when, in medical school, I happened to come across an article by Fred A. Whitehead, Bruce S. Liese, and Michael L. O'Dell most appropriately published in the *New York State Journal of Medicine* (Whitehead et al., 1990) where the authors clearly make the correct diagnosis. That is, they appreciate the diagnosis that Melville created for Bartleby. (The authors were from the Department of Family Practice, University of Kansas Medical Center in Kansas City, Missouri. Clearly, sometimes distance from place gives one the correct perspective!)

As Whitehead, Liese, and O'Dell note, Bartleby shows none of the positive symptoms of schizophrenia such as hallucinations, delusions, disordered speech, or behavior. Indeed, remember that, when visited by his former employer in jail, Bartleby is completely oriented to person and place, and speaks cogently and with insight into his condition. Bartleby does demonstrate some *negative symptoms* of schizophrenia such as alogia or pauci-alogia (lack of or very little speech), but these alone are not enough to diagnose schizophrenia by DSM-5 criteria. Bartleby certainly demonstrates social and occupational dysfunction, but if one looks at the DSM-5 criteria this is a feature of almost any psychiatric disorder or diagnosis.

In the DSM-5, catatonia can be a feature accompanying various diagnoses such as depression, schizophrenia, bipolar disorder, or others. A

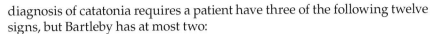

diagnosis of catatonia requires a patient have three of the following twelve signs, but Bartleby has at most two:

1. Catalepsy (i.e., passive induction of a posture held against gravity)
2. Waxy flexibility (i.e., slight and even resistance to positioning by examiner)
3. Stupor (no psychomotor activity; not actively relating to environment)
4. Agitation, not influenced by external stimuli
5. Mutism (i.e., no, or very little, verbal response [Note: not applicable if there is an established aphasia])
6. Negativism (i.e., opposing or not responding to instructions or external stimuli)
7. Posturing (i.e., spontaneous and active maintenance of a posture against gravity)
8. Mannerisms (i.e., odd caricature of normal actions)
9. Stereotypies (i.e., repetitive, abnormally frequent, non-goal directed movements)
10. Grimacing
11. Echolalia (i.e., mimicking another's speech)
12. Echopraxia (i.e., mimicking another's movements)

(In earlier versions of the DSM, catatonia was listed as a subtype of schizophrenia. DSM-5 contains only one significant change in the criteria for major depression[1].)

Comparison with Table 5.1 reveals Bartleby's diagnosis of severe major depression, not schizophrenia. Sadly, Bartleby's case ends as depression too often can, especially in a severe case such as this one, with a suicide.

Melville was a very complex individual, and depression was not unknown to him. One has to think that Bartleby comes somewhat from Melville's personal experience. This is an interesting question for further study.

TABLE 5.1 ❧ Diagnostic Criteria for Major Depression

A. Almost every day for at least two weeks, five of the following symptoms with at least one of the five being symptoms one or two:

1. Depressed mood most of the day, almost every day, indicated by your own subjective report or by the report of others. This mood might be characterized by sadness, emptiness, or hopelessness.

2. Markedly diminished interest or pleasure in all or almost all activities most of the day nearly every day

3. Significant weight loss when not dieting or weight gain

4. Inability to sleep or oversleeping nearly every day

5. Psychomotor agitation or retardation nearly every day

6. Fatigue or loss of energy nearly every day

7. Feelings of worthlessness or excessive or inappropriate guilt (which may be delusional) nearly every day

8. Diminished ability to think or concentrate, or indecisiveness, nearly every day

9. Recurrent thoughts of death (not just fear of dying), recurrent suicidal ideation without a specific plan, or a suicide attempt or a specific plan for committing suicide

B. Symptoms cause clinically significant distress or impairment in social, occupational, or other important areas of functioning.

C. The episode is not due to the effects of a substance or to a medical condition.

D. The occurrence is not better explained by schizoaffective disorder, schizophrenia, schizophreniform disorder, delusional disorder, or other specified and unspecified schizophrenia spectrum and other psychotic disorders.

E. There has never been a manic episode or a hypomanic episode.

(Reprinted with permission from the *Diagnostic and Statistical Manual of Mental Disorders, Fifth Edition,* © 2013. American Psychiatric Association.)

6

An Elementary Diagnosis

WE HAVE THUS FAR MAINLY DISCUSSED DSM-5 diagnoses in adults. One DSM-5 condition which first manifests in young children is autism. Autism is a complex condition still not well understood, and there can be a range of symptoms and severity. The core deficit seems to be in recognizing the emotions, feelings, and thoughts of others. Other features of autism can include low IQ and speech and other language problems. Due to the variation in symptoms and severity, the DSM 5 formally recognizes a spectrum of autism disorder (ASD).

Curiously, while ASD affects about 1% of school-age children (www. nichd.nih.gov/health/topics/autism/conditioninfo/Pages/at-risk.aspx), the first reports of autism were in the 1940s (Kanner, 1943; Asperger, 1944). But if ASD is a genetic disorder, as seems to be the case, how could such a common disease suddenly occur all across the world? I think that the recent description of ASD is likely not due to ASD being a new disease, but to a lack of reporting. Language difficulties in ASD would typically prevent patients from writing self-descriptions of the condition, and parents may not have brought ASD to the attention of clinicians and scientists. Also the complexity of ASD may have hindered an earlier description.

However, one end of the autism spectrum has very high functioning individuals. This portion is now known eponymously as Asperger's syndrome (Asperger, 1944). We can look to literature—in this case to the Sherlock Holmes stories (written by Sir Arthur Conan Doyle)—to find an Asperger's case study long before it's described in the medical literature.

Sherlock Holmes describes his older brother Mycroft in *The Adventure of the Bruce-Partington Plans* (Doyle, 1917) as follows:

> *"There has never been anything like it before, nor will be again. He has the tidiest and most orderly brain, with the greatest capacity for storing facts, of any man living. The same great powers which I have turned to the detection of crime he has used for this particular business. The conclusions of every department are passed to him, and he is the central exchange, the clearing-house, which makes out the balance. All other men are specialists, but his specialism is omniscience. We will suppose that a minister needs information as to a point which involves the Navy, India, Canada and the bimetallic question; he could get his separate advices from various departments upon each, but only Mycroft can focus them all, and say offhand how each factor would affect the other. They began by using him as a short-cut, a convenience; now he has made himself an essential. In that great brain of his everything is pigeon-holed and can be handed out in an instant."*

In *The Adventure of the Greek Interpreter* (Doyle, 1893), Sherlock Holmes again talks similarly about his brother Mycroft and also notes his highly regimented and unchanging daily routine. Mycroft is a co-founder of the Diogenes Club, a club that requires that, "No member is permitted to take the least notice of any other." The significance of this club rule is that there are kinds of behaviors—adherence to routines and avoidance of social interactions—often seen in individuals with Asperger's. Mycroft is also mentioned briefly in *The Final Problem* and *The Adventure of the Empty House*.

Besides Mycroft, Holmes mentions his family only two other times, but these are most interesting: Holmes notes that he and Mycroft are from a family of country squires (landowners) except for their grand-mother, whose brother was the French painter Émile Jean-Horace Vernet (1789–1863) (wikipedia.org/wiki/Horace_Vernet). Horace Vernet's father Carle Vernet (1758–1835), grandfather Claude-Joseph Vernet (1714–1789), and great-grandfather Antoine Vernet (1689–1753) were also painters. Thus, we know (within the context of the Holmes canon) who one of the great–great–great grandfathers of Sherlock and Mycroft was! There is a self-portrait of Horace Vernet (1835) at the Hermitage and a stunning portrait of Joseph Vernet by Louise Elisabeth Vigee Le Brun (1788) at the Louvre. So we have some idea what Holmes' ancestors looked like, though he did not specify which grandmother was the sister of Vernet.

Finally, in *The Adventure of the Norwood Builder* a physician named Verner, who was a distant relative of Sherlock Holmes, bought Watson's medical practice apparently at a premium price.

Both Sherlock Holmes (and Doyle) appreciated the centrality of genetics in the makeup of humans: The resolution of *The Hound of the Baskervilles* is centered on the physical resemblance of a character to the portrait of an unappreciated ancestor. Moreover, in *The Adventure of the Greek Interpreter*, Sherlock Holmes points out that both his and Mycroft's deductive powers are hereditary and "in the blood." Autism is now known to have a strong genetic etiologic component (www.nichd.nih.gov/health/topics/autism/conditioninfo/Pages/at-risk.aspx). If Asperger's genes are ever reliably known, and there are amenable descendants of Vernet, it would be interesting to learn if Horace Vernet had such DNA.

There have been many suggestions of a diagnosis of Asperger's syndrome for Sherlock based, for example, on his typical solitary and impersonal ways, as well as his intense, single-minded powers of concentration and exhaustive study of seeming minutia, such as soils and shoe tracks. With genetics now making the case elementary, I submit (Altschuler, 2013) that more than a half-century before Hans Asperger's description (Asperger, 1944), the syndrome ran in the Holmes family and affected both brothers.

The exclusion criteria and differential diagnosis for Asperger's include developmental delay or disorder (there is no evidence for this in either brother, in particular no evidence of language delay), and schizotypal and schizoid personality disorders. Neither brother exhibits the magical thinking of schizotypal personality disorder. And, though both brothers show schizoid tendencies, both can be most engaged and engaging when necessary.

Even further back in history, there are individuals who have had Asperger's. Neurologist Oliver Sacks (Sacks, 2001) showed quite convincingly that British physicist Henry Cavendish (1731–1810) most likely had Asperger's. Cavendish was a brilliant experimental and theoretical chemist and physicist, and his list of accomplishments and discoveries is impressive. He discovered hydrogen gas and, through careful experimentation, discovered that along with nitrogen and oxygen, air contained less than one percent of another substance. (It would be almost another century before William Ramsay and Lord Raleigh confirmed Cavendish's finding and named the substance argon.) In addition, Cavendish made the first measurement of the gravitational constant (G), finding a value within one percent of the modern one, and he discovered the inverse square law for the electrostatic force. He worked alone on experiments in a laboratory he built at his house, and instructed his servants to communicate with him only in writing. (Due to inheritance Cavendish was one of the richest men in England, yet he didn't seem to care about money.)

Examining literary and historical texts is an interesting way to study the prevalence of Asperger's in the past. For example, one could conceive of a project to look at all novels and stories published in a given year to ascertain the prevalence of Asperger's and autism spectrum disorder. As a matter of fact, John Donvan and Caren Zucker have recently shown that in an 1848 report to the Massachusetts legislature, Boston physician Samuel Gridley Howe (1801–1876), director of the Perkins Institution (now known as the Perkins School for the Blind), a school for children with blindness and other learning problems, provided examples of children with autism and Asperger's (Donovan and Zucker, 2016).

7

ADHD in a Seventeenth Century Dutch *Village School*

LIKE AUTISM SPECTRUM DISORDER (ASD), attention deficit hyperactivity disorder (ADHD) is a DSM disorder/diagnosis that typically first presents in children. Also like autism spectrum disorders, ADHD is now quite common—thought to affect 5–10% of school age children (more commonly boys) (Katragadda and Schubiner, 2007). Classification and diagnosis of ADHD has happened relatively recently. The first reports of ADHD in the medical literature are little more than a hundred years old (Still, 1902). Why did ADHD get explained in medical literature only in the last century? The answer may originate in our evolution away from a more agrarian society. When the world was more agrarian, ADHD could have been a beneficial, and indeed desired, trait to see in a male child: first the boy tends to one set of animals, then another, then the crops, then…. While I think the push and goals of universal childhood schooling (not farming) do not *cause* ADHD, it certainly unmasks the symptoms. In the context of formal schooling, the inclination to constantly move around from one activity to another is now considered a problem.

As with the other disorders we've discussed so far, we can look to literature and history to find examples of ADHD long before it appeared in the medical or scientific literature. And such examples can be found consistent with ADHD *not* being a new entity. We will also find a most interesting and beautiful surprise!

The DSM-5 criteria for ADHD are listed in Table 7.1. The DSM-5 (as its predecessor did) recognizes inattention and hyperactivity-impulsivity forms of ADHD. There can also be a mixed type where symptoms of both types are present for at least six months. (The presentation of ADHD in adults is different than in children, and as such, the DSM-5 has modified it's requirements so that an adult has to present five, not six, criteria.)

TABLE 7.1 Diagnostic Criteria for ADHD

A. A persistent pattern of inattention and/or hyperactivity-impulsivity that interferes with functioning or development, as characterized by (1) and/or (2):

   1. **Inattention:** Six (or more) of the following symptoms have persisted for at least 6 months to a degree that is inconsistent with developmental level and that negatively impacts directly on social and academic/occupational activities:

      Note: The symptoms are not solely a manifestation of oppositional behavior, defiance, hostility, or failure to understand tasks or instructions. For older adolescents and adults (age 17 and older), at least five symptoms are required.

      a. Often fails to give close attention to details or makes careless mistakes in schoolwork, at work, or during other activities (e.g., overlooks or misses details, work is inaccurate).

      b. Often has difficulty sustaining attention in tasks or play activities (e.g., has difficulty remaining focused during lectures, conversations, or lengthy reading).

      c. Often does not seem to listen when spoken to directly (e.g., mind seems elsewhere, even in the absence of any obvious distraction).

      d. Often does not follow through on instructions and fails to finish schoolwork, chores, or duties in the workplace (e.g., starts tasks but quickly loses focus and is easily sidetracked).

      e. Often has difficulty organizing tasks and activities (e.g., difficulty managing sequential tasks; difficulty keeping materials and belongings in order; messy, disorganized work; has poor time management; fails to meet deadlines).

      f. Often avoids, dislikes, or is reluctant to engage in tasks that require sustained mental effort (e.g., schoolwork or homework; for older adolescents and adults, preparing reports, completing forms, reviewing lengthy papers).

      g. Often loses things necessary for tasks or activities (e.g., school materials, pencils, books, tools, wallets, keys, paperwork, eyeglasses, mobile telephones).

      h. Is often easily distracted by extraneous stimuli (for older adolescents and adults, may include unrelated thoughts).

      i. Is often forgetful in daily activities (e.g., doing chores, running errands; for older adolescents and adults, returning calls, paying bills, keeping appointments).

   2. **Hyperactivity and impulsivity:** Six (or more) of the following symptoms have persisted for at least 6 months to a degree that is inconsistent with developmental level and that negatively impacts directly on social and academic/occupational activities:

      Note: The symptoms are not solely a manifestation of oppositional behavior, defiance, hostility, or a failure to understand tasks or instructions. For older adolescents and adults (age 17 and older), at least five symptoms are required.

TABLE 7.1 *(continued)*

a. Often fidgets with or taps hands or feet or squirms in seat.

b. Often leaves seat in situations when remaining seated is expected (e.g., leaves his or her place in the classroom, in the office or other workplace, or in other situations that require remaining in place).

c. Often runs about or climbs in situations where it is inappropriate. (**Note:** In adolescents or adults, may be limited to feeling restless.)

d. Often unable to play or engage in leisure activities quietly.

e. Is often "on the go," acting as if "driven by a motor" (e.g., is unable to be or uncomfortable being still for extended time, as in restaurants, meetings; may be experienced by others as being restless or difficult to keep up with).

f. Often talks excessively.

g. Often blurts out an answer before a question has been completed (e.g., completes people's sentences; cannot wait for turn in conversation).

h. Often has difficulty waiting his or her turn (e.g., while waiting in line).

i. Often interrupts or intrudes on others (e.g., butts into conversations, games, or activities; may start using other people's things without asking or receiving permission; for adolescents and adults, may intrude into or take over what others are doing).

B. Several inattentive or hyperactive-impulsive symptoms were present prior to age 12 years.

C. Several inattentive or hyperactive-impulsive symptoms are present in two or more settings (e.g., at home, school, or work; with friends or relatives; in other activities).

D. There is clear evidence that the symptoms interfere with, or reduce the quality of, social, academic, or occupational functioning.

E. The symptoms do not occur exclusively during the course of schizophrenia or another psychotic disorder and are not better explained by another mental disorder (e.g., mood disorder, anxiety disorder, dissociative disorder, personality disorder, substance intoxication or withdrawal).

(Reprinted with permission from the *Diagnostic and Statistical Manual of Mental Disorders, Fifth Edition,* © 2013. American Psychiatric Association.)

Thome and Jacobs (Thome and Jacobs, 2004) noted a description of the mixed inattentive and hyperactive subtype of ADHD in "The Story of Fidgety Philip" ('Zappel-Philipp') from the Second Edition (1846) of the children's book *Struwwelpeter* (Hoffmann, 1935) by German psychiatrist Heinrich Hoffmann (1809–1894):

But Philip he did not mind
His father who was so kind.
He wriggled
And giggled,

And then, I declare,
Swung backward and forward
And tilted his chair …

Auster (1999) noticed the inattentive subtype of ADHD in a child who could not concentrate and learn his lessons despite hundreds of attempts, described more than 100 years ago in the Babylonian Talmud: "'What', the Master asked, 'is the matter today?' 'From the moment', the pupil replied, 'the Master was told that there was a religious matter to be attended to I could not concentrate my thoughts, for at every moment I imagined, Now the Master will get up or Now the Master will get up.'"

Veering away from literary works, briefly, an interpretation (Kast and Altschuler, 2008) of the painting *The Village School* (c. 1670) (Figure 7.1) by Dutch master Jan Steen (c. 1626–1679) clearly illustrates that ADHD is an old disease.

A modern diagnosis of ADHD (see Table 7.1) hyperactivity subtype, requires that six of nine criteria (six hyperactivity criteria and three impulsivity criteria) be met. The children in the painting illustrate all six of the hyperactivity criteria: (1) often fidgets with hands or feet or squirms in their seat; (2) often leaves their seat in classroom or in other situations in

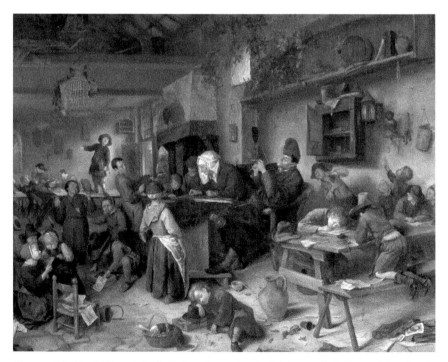

Figure 7.1 *The Village School.* By Jan Steen (c. 1670). National Gallery of Scotland.

which remaining seated is expected; (3) often runs about or climbs excessively in situations in which it is inappropriate (in adolescents or adults this may be limited to subjective feelings of restlessness); (4) often has difficulty playing or engaging in leisure activities quietly; (5) is often "on the go" or often acts as if "driven by a motor"; and (6) often talks excessively. The three impulsivity criteria—blurting out answers, not waiting one's turn and interrupting others—cannot be met, but only because there is not sufficient order in the school to interrupt! These criteria are evident in children under 7 years of age, clearly cause academic dysfunction, and are not associated with other psychiatric or developmental disorders.

Despite the children in the painting meeting criteria for the hyperactivity subtype of ADHD, we are still compelled to consider, as when making a diagnosis in medicine, other causes of the same symptoms. Does the painting represent something other than ADHD, in particular the normal state of childhood with "boys being boys?" Steen's painting has the wonderful ambiguity of great art, and an interpretation of the painting as exaggerated play certainly comes to mind when looking at it. However, contrast with another Steen painting (Figure 7.2) from approximately 5 years earlier, also (confusingly) now known as *The Village School*, provides perhaps the strongest evidence that something is seriously wrong

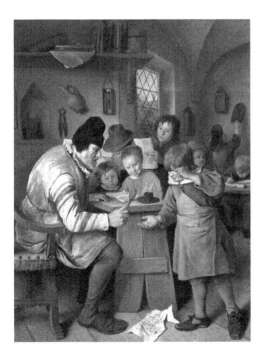

Figure 7.2 *The Village School*. By Jan Steen (c. 1665). National Gallery of Ireland.

and amiss in the 1670 painting. Indeed, all the children (except one) in the 1665 painting are impeccably behaved, and the child who is being punished seems to have insight and regret for his transgression, or at least for his punishment!

Finally, we must also consider that the 1670 painting simply represent Steen's "style" and not ADHD. Indeed, a certain amount of mayhem is not uncommon in Steen's paintings, for example as is seen in his So the Old Sing, So Twitter the Young (c. 1665, now at The Mauritshuis). However, as in this painting and others by Steen, the mayhem is circumscribed in a way that the activity in *The Village School* (1670) is not.

Furthermore, disorder in Steen's paintings is typically associated with drunkenness that is of course not found in the *The Village School*.

Even more remarkable, Jan Steen's painting *The Village School* (1670) is the oldest known (so far) depiction or description of the hyperactivity subtype of ADHD. Like all great art it is provocative and, as such, not only illustrates this particular disorder, but also introduces some ambiguity as it charges us to consider the boundary and distinction between ADHD and normal childhood. Steen's painting, combined with observations of the mixed and inattentive subtypes of ADHD in literature and history (Auster, 1999; Hoffmann, 1935; Thome and Jacobs, 2004) show that ADHD is not a disease new to the 20th and 21st centuries. It also is most interesting that two of the three historic cases are in school settings.

8

Disease in the Hundred Acre Wood
Pediatric Psychiatric Disease in Literature

SO FAR WE HAVE TALKED ABOUT several psychiatric diseases that start in childhood, as well as several that begin in adulthood. But what about the stereotypical "adult" DSM-5 diagnoses like depression or bipolar disorder ("manic-depression")? Can children get these diseases?

One night, when I was in medical school during the inpatient portion of my pediatrics rotation, we admitted a child for a streaking rash spreading up his arm. The team's working diagnosis was a type of spider bite that can lead to infections. These bites infect the skin and can become so severe that dead flesh may need to be surgically removed or, in the worst cases, limb amputation may be necessary to stop the spread of the infection. The night the child came in, one of the doctors remembered that he had been admitted with another spider bite just two months previously. What is the chance of two spider bites in two months? The doctor suggested "something else must be going on."

I was prompted to go over the patient's history again. When in doubt, as it is taught, recheck the history and physical examination. The thorough history and physical examination revealed that the patient had a longstanding diagnosis of bipolar disorder, potentially with psychotic features. History taken at his previous admission showed that the patient was supposed to be on a lot of powerful medications for these disorders. However, as blood levels of the medications at the current and prior admissions showed, he had likely not been taking the prescribed medication. I pointed this out and suggested that the manic phase of bipolar disorder could have caused the patient to inject something into his arm that was potentially mimicking a spider bite and causing his current problem. Indeed, subsequent interviews with the patient and family revealed that in fact there was no spider bite causing this admission. Eventually the infection was controlled but not without a significant number of days on antibiotics as well as surgery to remove dead skin that left permanent scars and was extremely painful.

Could full-strength doses of all of his medication have prevented the actions that might have caused the problem on this admission? At the time it was not necessarily common practice to treat, or often diagnose, children with "adult" disease.

But children are increasingly being diagnosed with the full panoply of adult diseases. Some cynics say that this is fueled by the drug companies wanting to sell more medicines to kids. As in all previous chapters, let's see if, and how, great literature can illuminate our understanding of adult psychiatric disease in kids. It turns out that A. A. Milne's Hundred Acre Wood, of all places, is a veritable laboratory to study DSM-5 diagnoses in children. The consideration—by doctors other than myself—of psychiatric disease found in the characters in *Winnie-the-Pooh* (1926) began to appear in print in December, 2000.

The Christmas issue of the *British Medical Journal* (*BMJ*) is a double issue that contains articles less serious than the typical fare in the *BMJ* the rest of the year, including articles about medicine and science in culture, society, art, history, and literature. The *Canadian Medical Journal* (*CMJ*) does so as well. Around Christmas 2000, I saw a news story about a paper published in the *CMJ* describing disease in the Hundred Acre Wood. The authors of the article, Sarah Shea and colleagues from the Department of Pediatrics at Dalhousie University, Halifax, NS, have tongue-in-cheek diagnoses for a variety of Milne's characters (Shea et al., 2000).

While Shea et al. were tongue in cheek, another physician was less so about diagnosing the characters in the Hundred Acre Wood. Indeed, five months after Shea et al.'s article was published, Leo Bastiaens (www.cmaj.ca/content/163/12/1557.full/reply#cmaj_e_78), a psychiatrist from Pittsburgh, wrote in saying that for a decade before Shea et al.'s paper, he had been lecturing on the psychiatric pathology in the Hundred Acre Wood, which he noticed while reading the series to his children. Though scooped in print by Shea et al., Bastiaens was helpful in refining many of the diagnoses of Shea and her colleagues. It is interesting to read the Winnie-the-Pooh books by A.A. Milne, *Winnie-the-Pooh* (London: Methuen; 1926) and *The House at Pooh Corner* (London: Methuen; 1928), and decide what you think the diagnoses for the characters are (it is also worthwhile to look at the interactions among the characters). Table 8.1 lists Shea's and Bastiaens' diagnoses; I personally think that Bastiaens is essentially correct. The DSM-5 criteria for these diagnoses are given elsewhere in the book.

In a number of ways, these diagnoses stand out and have a lot to teach us. Bastiaens suggests a diagnosis of a disease called Prader-Willi syn-

TABLE 8.1 Shea and Bastiaens *Winnie the Pooh* Character Diagnoses

Character	Life Stressors	Shea et al.	Bastiaens
Winnie the Pooh	—	ADHD[a]; inattentive subtype OCD (provisional diagnosis); low IQ; poor diet; obesity; binge eating	Prader-Willi Syndrome
Piglet	Failure to thrive	General anxiety disorder (GAD)[b]	—
Eeyore	Traumatic tail amputation; housing problems	Dysthymic disorder[c]	Major depression[d]
Rabbit	—	Narcissistic personality disorder	Obsessive compulsive disorder (OCD)[e]
Owl	Housing problems	Reading disorder; narcissistic personality disorder[f]	Dyslexia[g]
Tigger	—	ADHD; hyperactivity-impulsivity subtype	ADHD combined type
Kanga	Single; unemployed parent; overprotective of child	—	Separation anxiety disorder[h]
Roo	Single-parent household	—	Separation anxiety disorder
Christopher Robin	Lack of parental supervision; possible educational problems	Gender identity disorder[i]	—

a. For ADHD criteria, see Chapter 6.
b. For GAD criteria, see Chapter 8 Notes, Table 1.
c. For Dysthymia criteria, see Chapter 8 Notes, Table 2.
d. For Major Depression criteria, see Chapter 5.
e. For OCD criteria, see Chapter 8 Notes, Table 3.
f. For Narcissistic Personality Disorder, see Chapter 8 Notes, Table 4.
g. For Dyslexia criteria, see Chapter 9.
h. For Separation Anxiety Disorder, see Chapter 8 Notes, Table 5.
i. For Gender Identity Disorder, see Chapter 8 Notes, Table 6. In the DSM-5, gender identity disorder has been renamed gender dysphoria.

drome for Pooh, rather than the dual occurring psychiatric diagnoses ADHD and OCD that Shea et al. make. Shea et al. also diagnose Winnie with borderline intellectual functioning (e.g., Pooh's own comments that he has "very little brain"), and obesity and binge eating. In fact, these are all features of Prader-Willi syndrome, along with others that Bastiaens points out in Pooh: insatiability despite his overeating, a somewhat overly cheerful manner, and the small chin and hypogonadism of Prader-Willi. The numerous excellent illustrations of Pooh by Ernest Shepard show Pooh with no pants, but no sexual development either. (Fascinatingly, the overeating and insatiability of Pooh was previously noted long ago [Gault, 1965]). Pooh's case illustrates that in making a DSM-5 diagnosis, one must always keep "pure" medical or genetic causes of symptoms in mind.

Prader-Willi is a genetically complex disorder associated with microdeletions of genes on chromosome 15. The eponym for the disease comes from a 1956 paper describing a series of patients with the disorder (Prader et al., 1956). In 1981, chromosome 15 was located as the place of microdeletions in the disorder. Now it is accepted that Prader-Willi syndrome results from a failure of certain modifications of genes transmitted on chromosome 15 from the father to the baby. Interestingly, a possible case of Prader-Willi was described by Hopkins in 1861, and the first complete description given in 1864 by John Langdon Down (for whom "Down's syndrome" was named in 1961).

An odd feature of Prader-Willi syndrome is that, despite all of their deficits, Prader-Willi individuals are typically supernormal (better than normals) at jigsaw puzzles (Dykens, 2002). Milne may have noticed and alluded to it in Chapter 1 of *The House at Pooh Corner* in which Pooh helps build a house for Eeyore.

Why do the Pooh books hold such appeal for children and their parents, despite the high and omnipresent burden of psychiatric disease and developmental pathology? It seems to me that the biggest draw of the books is Pooh himself. His likability may be fueled by the "extra" childlike characteristics that Prader-Willi can endow on a fictional character. Indeed, my teacher Stephen Jay Gould discussed the "evolution" of Mickey Mouse over the years and noted a positive correlation between Mickey's increasing popularity and more childlike features for Mickey such as a rounded face, compared with his initial angular one (Gould, 1980).

A deeper issue to consider is whether a number of parents and even children are also drawn to these books because the portrayal of illness adds complexity and depth to the characters and plot. Overall, the characters try to help one another with their problems. In *Winnie-the-Pooh*, Chapter 6, the animals have a birthday party for Eeyore to cheer him up; in Chapter 7 the animals try to help Kanga and Roo with their separation anxiety; and in Chapter 1 of *The House at Pooh Corner*, Pooh and Piglet build a house for Eeyore.

There is so much psychopathology in the books—affecting each and every character—that it seems hard to believe that there was not some intentionality on the part of Milne. Why did Milne incorporate so much psychiatric disease in *Winnie-the-Pooh*? It would be interesting to look into this question as well as Milne's history, to see if any of the characters and/or their diseases derived from his history.

9

Moving and Sleeping with Dickens and Dracula

CHARLES DICKENS WAS NOT ONLY one of the greatest writers of all time, he was also one of the most observant. Dickens was an astute observer of the human condition in all arenas—social and vocational—and of people in all strata of society. Thus, perhaps not surprisingly, Dickens was also a keen observer and chronicler of medical conditions, as discussed in a most excellent and entertaining article—available for free access online—by the British neurologist Lord Russell Brain in the 1955 Christmas issue of *British Medical Journal* (Brain, 1955). Two areas of particular interest for Dickens were movement and sleep disorders. Many of Dickens characters had DSM-5 diagnoses in these categories.

Cosnett pointed out that in Dickens' 1857 novel, *Little Dorit* the character Jeremiah Flintwinch has focal dystonia with torticollis (Cosnett, 1991). That is, Flintwich typically has his neck in a twisted and odd position. This is a neurologic disease and not a DSM diagnosis, but such abnormal positionings can also be symptoms of medications used to treat schizophrenia. So Dickens' vivid descriptions are often relevant to discussions of DSM disorders. Cosnett further notes that Mr. Pancks, another character in the same novel, had multiple ticks and inappropriate vocalizations, which would be consistent with a modern diagnosis of Tourette's syndrome. These character descriptions seem so realistic and vivid that Cosnett says, and I agree, that Dickens must have modeled them on people that he knew. Interestingly, this depiction of Tourette's syndrome came nearly thirty years before George Gilles de la Tourette's classic paper on the disease (Gilles de la Tourette, 1885)! (However, another French neurologist Jacque Itard published a description of what we would recognize today as Tourette's syndrome in 1825 [Itard, 1825]—a decade before Dickens' novel. More examples of movement disorders in Dickens can be found in Perkin, 1996.)

Possibly an even more prescient Dickensian diagnosis was noted by Larner (Larner, 2002): In a rarely read Dickens work, *The Lazy Tour of Two Idle Apprentices* (Dickens and Collins, 1857), there may be the first description of a disease known as progressive supranuclear palsy (PSP). In *The Lazy Tour*, two characters who clearly represent Dickens and his friend Wilkie Collins tour northern England. At an inn in Lancaster, the character representing Dickens notices and describes a most interesting individual:

> *A chilled, slow, earthy, fixed old man. A cadaverous man of measured speech. An old man who seemed as unable to wink, as if his eyelids had been nailed to his forehead. An old man whose eyes—two spots of fire— had no more motion that [sic] if they had been connected with the back of his skull by screws driven through it, and rivetted and bolted outside, among his grey hair.*

> *He had come in and shut the door, and he now sat down. He did not bend himself to sit, as other people do, but seemed to sink bolt upright, as if in water, until the chair stopped him.*

(Dickens and Collins, 1857)

Now, the definitive description of PSP was given in 1964 by Steele, Richardson and Olszewski. Typically, PSP is thought of as a Parkinson "plus" syndrome. That is, patients with PSP exhibit symptoms of an unsteady gait (requiring a stooped posture in Parkinson's), bradykinesia and slow movements, as well as other defining features such as ophthalmoplegia or lack of movement of the eyes, lid retraction and axial dystonia, or unusual postures of the spine. As Larner notes, the character meets most of these criteria, except for an important one, an unsteady gait. Thus, it is not a slam dunk that this is the oldest description of PSP. But, given the vivid, detailed description, the character is likely to mimic a real person that Dickens saw at some point. So even if this is not the first description of PSP—a century ahead of the medical profession—maybe Dickens noticed a disease or condition we still don't fully appreciate. PSP is not a DSM diagnosis, but the DSM-5 includes neurocogntive disorders associated with Parkinson's disease, Huntington's disease, HIV infection, and other neurologic diseases.

In terms of sleep, as Cosnett points out (Cosnett, 1992), Dickens seems to have described the full DSM-5 panoply of problems and conditions that can occur in the complete cycle of sleep from falling asleep to waking up: insomnia; hypnagogic hallucinations—hallucinations one can have just before falling asleep—to possibly the first description of restless leg syndrome[1]; nightmares; and sleep walking. As well, in *Oliver Twist* (1837–1839) Dickens' description of sleep paralysis—paralysis that happens while sleeping, where one is thinking and wanting to move, but cannot—predated the "official" (Mitchell, 1876) description by nearly 40 years.

In medical circles Dickens' character fat Joe in *The Posthumous Papers of the Pickwick Club* (1837) is very well known for his syndrome of obesity and daytime somnolence (Burwell et al., 1956). Today this Pickwickian syndrome is usually associated with an increasing common condition of not only obesity and daytime somnolence, but also apneic episodes (obstructive sleep apnea, or, OSA) in which sufferers experience multiple short periods of sleep during which they can literally stop breathing hundreds of times. Dickens mentions no apneic episodes for fat Joe, though as Cosnett points out (Cosnett, 1992) Dickens certainly is aware of this symptom as it is clearly described in characters such as Mr. Willet in *Barnaby Rudge* (1867).

Amazingly, even centuries before Dickens, Shakespeare describes the full modern day "standard" obesity/hypoventilation/daytime somnolence/sleep apnea syndrome in Fallstaff. It is a marvel befitting the poet that he accomplishes this description in only two lines:

Peto: Falstaff! Fast asleep behind the arras, and snorting like a horse.

Prince: Hark, how hard he fetches breath. Search his pockets.

(Henry IV, Part 1 Act 2, Scene 4)

OSA is a condition that should be considered more often in historical and literary records. Most people with large necks and significant snoring probably have the condition. An interesting article by Margolis (Margolis, 2000) suggested that the great composer Johannes Brahms (1833–1897), who had quite a stout neck and was known to be a loud and inveterate snorer, may have had OSA. Could this have influenced Brahms to write his famous lullaby?

Why Dickens' great interest in sleep? Cosnett notes that Dickens' interest into diseases of sleep may be related to his own self-described insomnia and his turning this potential negative into a positive: Dickens used long walks at night to try to treat his insomnia, and he also used the time he was walking to plan his books and stories.

More about sleep diagnoses can be found in other literary works. For example, there is sleep walking by Lady Macbeth in *Macbeth*, which will be discussed in more detail in Chapter 11, *Shakespeare*.

Along with descriptions and observations of many disorders of sleep and also deficits from stroke and other neurodegenerative diseases affecting older folks, Dickens has one of the earliest and clearest descriptions of a DSM-5 diagnosis that typically shows itself in the first years of school—dyslexia. In the 1992 Christmas issue of the *Lancet*, N. M. Jacoby (Jacoby, 1992) describes a case of dyslexia to be found in Mr. Krook from Dickens' 1853 novel *Bleak House*.

Krook has the most severe form of dyslexia, known as word blindness. In Chapter XIV Esther Summerson describes a tour Mr. Krook gave her guardian, John Jarndyce, of his house:

> At last we came into the back part of the shop. Here on the head of an empty barrel stood on end, were an ink bottle, some old stamps of pens, and some dirty playbills; and, against the wall were pasted several large printed alphabets in several plain hands.

> "What are you doing here?" asked my guardian.

> "Trying to learn myself to read and write," said Krook.

> "And how do you get on?"

> "Slow. Bad," returned the old man, impatiently. "It's hard at my time of life."

> "It would be easier to be taught by some one," said my guardian.

Later, in Chapter XXXII, Tony Jobling and William Guppy are discussing whether or not Mr. Krook could read some letters from which they hope to profit:

> "Tony," says Mr. Guppy after considering a little with his legs crossed, "he can't read yet can he?"

> "Read!" He'll never read. He can make all the letters separately; and he knows most of them separately when he sees them; he has got on that much under me; but he can't put them together. He's too old to acquire the knack of it now—and too drunk."

> "Tony," says Mr. Guppy uncrossing and recrossing his legs, "How do you suppose he spelt out that name of Hawdon?"

> "He never spelt it out. You know what a curious power of eye he has and how he used to employ himself in copying things by eye alone. He imitated it—evidently from the direction of a letter; and asked me what it meant."

This description by Dickens predates by decades published descriptions of the disease in the medical literature. Most surely Dickens must have personally observed a child or an adult with the condition.

Even in mild forms, dyslexia remains a significant problem today without simple treatments. Dickens' description clearly illustrates the hurdles that need to be overcome.

Medicine and The Count

Near the end of my internship year I started reading *Dracula* (1897), Bram Stoker's (1847–1912) gripping tale. During the last month of my internship at Brooklyn Hospital Center, I was the night float, and strange things happen at hospitals at night. Brooklyn Hospital dates from the middle of the Nineteenth Century and is one of the older hospitals in the country. Some parts of the hospital still remained from early days and sometimes, when looking around a corner, one almost felt the earlier time present, if only for a second.

Interestingly, some years previously (Heick, 1992; Gomez-Alonso, 1998) it had been suggested that the vampire legend in general, which dated from about the seventeenth century, was inspired by rabies. Indeed, there are many crucial similarities between vampirism and rabies: For example, both are infectious—a bite from a vampire turns one into a vampire, just as a bite from a rabid animal can give another animal or person rabies. Frothing at the mouth, hypersexual behavior, biting, and general nocturnal phase activity are other features of vampirism that are often shared by rabid animals or people. The rabies virus takes a remarkable course, traveling up the peripheral nerves of the body to eventually reach the brain. There the virus infects the limbic system of the brain, one of the oldest, evolutionarily speaking, portions of the brain. The limbic system controls ancient and basic functions such as aggression, sexual activity, an individual's response to light, sleep-wake cycles, and salivary secretions. In this way, the virus ingeniously secures its own propagation and survival by causing a rabid animal to be aggressive enough to bite another animal, thereby transmitting the virus via copious oral secretions.

Another similarity between vampirism and rabies includes a predominance of dogs and wolves as transmitting animals. As well, rabid animals were common in central Europe in the late seventeenth century when vampire legends originated.

But in *Dracula,* Stoker goes far beyond local legends and myths, with medicine holding a prominent place in the action. For example, blood transfusions, diagnosis-based treatment, and the physicians David Ferrier (1843–1928), and Jean-Martin Charcot (1825–1893) are featured in the story. Also, two important characters in the book, John Seward and Professor Abraham Van Helsing, are physicians. This is not incidental or coincidental: Stoker spent orders of many times longer on *Dracula* than on any of his other literary projects—six years compared with a couple of months—reading widely at places such as the British Library for background for his book.

Bram Stoker's *Dracula* (1897) is a gripping tale that also has a few sleepwalking characters, perhaps not surprising given the nocturnal focus of *Dracula.* However, Stoker provides us with the first known discussion of hereditary somnambulism (sleepwalking) (Altschuler, 2003). Lucy Westenra—who, after being bitten by Count Dracula and becoming a vampire is eventually killed—had a long habit of sleepwalking. Furthermore, Lucy's mother, Mrs. Westenra, tells Mina Murray "... that her husband, Lucy's father, had the same habit [sleep-walking], that he would get up in the night and dress himself and go out, if he were not stopped." Thus, sleepwalking runs in the Westenra family (Altschuler, 2003). The next description of a hereditary component of somnambulism was not described again for nearly a half-century later (Davis, Hayes, Dirman, 1942). More recently (Kales et al., 1980), we can continue to find a hereditary component in somnambulism. But so far, no gene for somnambulism has been found.

Besides being an author, Bram Stoker graduated from Trinity College, Dublin with honors in mathematics, and worked as a civil servant and a manager for stage actors. "Bram" is short for Abraham, and one suspects that Stoker found himself in the eccentric, eclectic, and peripatetic genius Professor Van Helsing, who has not only an MD but also a DPh, and a DLit, and is a lawyer.

10

PTSD: A Continuing Saga of Many Wars and *Two Cities*

IN 1914, A FRENCH PHYSICIAN REPORTED on four soldiers with "battle hypnosis" (Milian, 1915). In 1915, a British physician reported on three soldiers who suffered "loss of memory, vision, smell and taste" (Myers, 1915), describing the condition as "shell shock." In 1917, a German psychiatrist, Robert Gaupp, described the symptoms of sudden muteness, deafness, and inability to stand or walk (Kaufmann, 1916) in soldiers. All of the above were considered symptoms of "shell shock," and were present in many soldiers who fought in WWI (Salmon, 1917). Similar symptoms were present in soldiers in WWII (Grinker and Spiegel, 1945), though often different names such as "war neuroses" or "operational fatigue" were used to describe them.

In 1952, symptoms such as shell shock or war neuroses were listed in the DSM-I in the category of "gross stress reaction." Strangely, this category was removed from the DSM-II. The experiences of numerous war veterans, including many U.S. Vietnam War veterans, and also the recognition that posttraumatic symptoms can be experienced not only by war veterans, but by individuals who have experienced traumatic events such as a sexual assault or natural disaster (symptoms can also be experienced by loved ones or caregivers of individuals who have experienced a traumatic event [Clawson et al., 2013]), led to the current diagnosis of posttraumatic stress disorder (PTSD), which appeared in the DSM-III (Bentley, 2005). The DSM-5 criteria for PTSD are listed in Table 10.1.

For his medical school dissertation, Swiss physician Johannes Hofer (1669–1752) described the concept of "nostalgia" (1688; University of Basel). Hofer's definition included melancholy, incessant thinking of home, disturbed sleep or insomnia, weakness, loss of appetite, anxiety, cardiac palpitations, stupor, and fever. Thousands of soldiers in the U.S. Civil War were diagnosed with "nostalgia." In 1871, Jacob Mendez DaCosta

TABLE 10.1 Diagnostic Criteria for Posttraumatic Stress Disorder

Note: The following criteria apply to adults, adolescents, and children older than 6 years. For children 6 years and younger, see corresponding criteria below.

A. Exposure to actual or threatened death, serious injury, or sexual violence in one (or more) of the following ways:

1. Directly experiencing the traumatic event(s).

2. Witnessing, in person, the event(s) as it occurred to others.

3. Learning that the traumatic event(s) occurred to a close family member or close friend. In cases of actual or threatened death of a family member or friend, the event(s) must have been violent or accidental.

4. Experiencing repeated or extreme exposure to aversive details of the traumatic event(s) (e.g., first responders collecting human remains; police officers repeatedly exposed to details of child abuse).

Note: Criterion A4 does not apply to exposure through electronic media, television, movies, or pictures, unless this exposure is work related.

B. Presence of one (or more) of the following intrusion symptoms associated with the traumatic event(s), beginning after the traumatic event(s) occurred:

1. Recurrent, involuntary, and intrusive distressing memories of the traumatic event(s).

Note: In children older than 6 years, repetitive play may occur in which themes or aspects of the traumatic event(s) are expressed.

2. Recurrent distressing dreams in which the content and/or affect of the dream are related to the traumatic event(s).

Note: In children, there may be frightening dreams without recognizable content.

3. Dissociative reactions (e.g., flashbacks) in which the individual feels or acts as if the traumatic event(s) were recurring. (Such reactions may occur on a continuum, with the most extreme expression being a complete loss of awareness of present surroundings.)

Note: In children, trauma-specific reenactment may occur in play.

4. Intense or prolonged psychological distress at exposure to internal or external cues that symbolize or resemble an aspect of the traumatic event(s).

5. Marked physiological reactions to internal or external cues that symbolize or resemble an aspect of the traumatic event(s).

C. Persistent avoidance of stimuli associated with the traumatic event(s), beginning after the traumatic event(s) occurred, as evidenced by one or both of the following:

1. Avoidance of or efforts to avoid distressing memories, thoughts, or feelings about or closely associated with the traumatic event(s).

2. Avoidance of or efforts to avoid external reminders (people, places, conversations, activities, objects, situations) that arouse distressing memories, thoughts, or feelings about or closely associated with the traumatic event(s).

TABLE 10.1 (*continued*)

D. Negative alterations in cognitions and mood that are associated with the traumatic event(s), beginning or worsening after the traumatic event(s) occurred, as evidenced by two (or more) of the following:

   1. Inability to remember an important aspect of the traumatic event(s) (typically due to dissociative amnesia and not to other factors such as head injury, alcohol, or drugs).

   2. Persistent and exaggerated negative beliefs or expectations about oneself, others, or the world (e.g., "I am bad," "No one can be trusted," "The world is completely dangerous," "My whole nervous system is permanently ruined").

   3. Persistent, distorted cognitions about the cause or consequences of the traumatic event(s) that lead the individual to blame himself/herself or others.

   4. Persistent negative emotional state (e.g., fear, horror, anger, guilt, or shame).

   5. Markedly diminished interest or participation in significant activities.

   6. Feelings of detachment or estrangement from others.

   7. Persistent inability to experience positive emotions (e.g., inability to experience happiness, satisfaction, or loving feelings).

E. Marked alterations in arousal and reactivity associated with the traumatic event(s), beginning or worsening after the traumatic event(s) occurred, as evidenced by two (or more) of the following:

   1. Irritable behavior and angry outbursts (with little or no provocation) typically expressed as verbal or physical aggression toward people or objects.

   2. Reckless or self-destructive behavior.

   3. Hypervigilance.

   4. Exaggerated startle response.

   5. Problems with concentration.

   6. Sleep disturbance (e.g., difficulty falling or staying asleep or restless sleep).

F. Duration of the disturbance (Criteria B, C, D, and E) is more than 1 month.

G. The disturbance causes clinically significant distress or impairment in social, occupational, or other important areas of functioning.

H. The disturbance is not attributable to the physiological effects of a substance (e.g., medication, alcohol) or another medical condition.

(Reprinted with permission from the *Diagnostic and Statistical Manual of Mental Disorders, Fifth Edition*, © 2013. American Psychiatric Association.)

described a constellation of symptoms in soldiers often occurring together—chest-thumping (tachycardia/palpitations), anxiety, and breathlessness—referred to as "soldier's heart" (DaCosta, 1871).

Another early name for PTSD was described by John Erichsen as "railway spine": a syndrome of posttraumatic mental symptoms in individuals who had survived railroad accidents which were not uncommon during this time (Erichsen, 1867).

The history of the human race is one of war, and PTSD seems to accompany all wars, so we would expect to find descriptions of PTSD throughout our written history. A problem in finding such evidence is that, as time recedes, there is less and less textual evidence and only a fraction of texts survive. Nevertheless, there are some hints of PTSD many centuries ago and in diverse geographic locations—the ancient Near East (Abdul-Hamid and Hughes, 2014) and the Indian subcontinent (Jayatunge, 2010), for example. The clearest description of PTSD from the past is an account from Mesopotamia more than four thousand years ago in which Ezra noted (Ezra, 2001) that a cuneiform tablet (Fluckiger-Hawker, 1999) described the Sumerian King Urnamma's death by battle (c. 2040 BCE) and its consequences, including a description of PTSD.

> *From the [... the...] was [...] evenly in/on the land. [The...] struck, the palace(s) was collapsed. [The...] spread panic rapidly among its Black-headed who dwelt there. [The...] established its abandoned places in Sumer. In its vast [...] cities are destroyed, the people are seized with panic. Evil came upon Ur...They weep bitter tears in their broad squares where merriment had reigned. With their bliss (fullness) having come to an end, the people do not sleep soundly.*

Great writers were aware of the disease as well, and literary "cases" go back in time. Huber and te Wildt make an interesting case that Dr. Manette from Dickens' *A Tale of Two Cities* experiences dissociative traumatic re-experiences in the context of PTSD (Huber and te Wildt, 2005). But remarkably (though is this word ever needed or warranted with regard to the Bard?) Shakespeare has a full and complete description of PTSD in *Henry IV*, Part 1 (1598) nearly a century earlier than Hofer!

An important character in the play is Henry Percy ("Hotspur") who, with his family, helped King Henry IV wrest the throne from Richard II and then, in extensive battles, fights on behalf of Henry, successfully defeating a Scottish rebellion. Later, Hotspur crosses purposes with King Henry and is eventually defeated in solo combat by Henry's son Hal, the future King Henry V.

In Act 2, Scene 3, Hotspur's wife Kate gives the following monologue to and about him (PTSD associated signs and symptoms are noted to the side [Shay, 2013]):

O, my good lord, why are you thus alone? [social withdrawal]

For what offence have I this fortnight been [random rage at family]

A banish'd woman from my Harry's bed? [sexual disinterest/dysfunction]

Tell me, sweet lord, what is't that takes from thee

Thy stomach, pleasure and thy golden sleep? [loss of interest, insomnia]

Why dost thou bend thine eyes upon the earth, [depression]

And start so often when thou sit'st alone? [hyperactive startle reaction]

Why hast thou lost the fresh blood in thy cheeks;

And given my treasures and my rights of thee

To thick-eyed musing and curst melancholy?

In thy faint slumbers I by thee have watch'd, [fragmented, vigilant sleep]

And heard thee murmur tales of iron wars; [traumatic dreams, reliving episodes of combat]

Speak terms of manage [horsemanship] to thy bounding steed;

Cry 'Courage! to the field!' And thou hast talk'd

Of sallies and retires, of trenches, tents,

Of palisadoes, frontiers, parapets,

Of basilisks, of cannon, culverin,

Of prisoners' ransom and of soldiers slain,

And all the currents of a heady fight.

Thy spirit within thee hath been so at war,

And thus hath so bestirr'd thee in thy sleep,

That beads of sweat have stood upon thy brow [night sweats]

Like bubbles in a late-disturbed stream;

And in thy face strange motions have appear'd,

Such as we see when men restrain their breath

On some great sudden hest. O, what portents are these?

Some heavy business hath my lord in hand,

And I must know it, else he loves me not.

Recently, I found (Altschuler, 2016) a previously undescribed form of PTSD, one that can have important consequences for our modern society and, also, likely did in the past. I found the case in the memoir of Robert Gates (Gates, 2014). In late 2011, Gates abruptly resigned as United States Secretary of Defense after serving in the position for four and a half years under two Presidents of different political parties. In the Author's Note to his 2014 memoir, *Duty*, Gates comments, "Toward the end of my time in office, I could barely speak to them [soldiers] or about them without being overcome with emotion. Early in my fifth year, I came to believe my determination to protect them …was clouding my judgment and diminishing my usefulness to the president …." In the book, Gates noted that "the hardest part of being secretary for me was visiting the wounded in hospitals … and it got harder each time." In reflecting (on the second to last page of the book) Gates writes, "… in my mind's eye I could see them [injured soldiers] lying awake, alone, in the hours before dawn, confronting their pain and their broken dreams and shattered lives. I would wake in the night, think back to a wounded soldier or Marine I had seen … and in my imagination, I would put myself in his hospital room and I would hold him to my chest, to comfort him … so my answer to the young soldier's question … about what kept me awake at night: he did."

We see that Gates has ongoing and longstanding recurrent recollections, dreams and awakenings about the injuries of soldiers under his command. These caused a significant vocational disturbance—he had to retire from his job! If these recollections were about trauma he had personally experienced, Gates would meet criteria for posttraumatic stress disorder (PTSD). As best is known, Gates personally did not experience such trauma, so his feelings and emotions are solely induced by trauma sustained by his subordinates. Gates' form of PTSD is unlike PTSD by proxy in caregivers or loved ones of the individual who experienced a trauma because, in this case, PTSD is being experienced by the person who ordered the traumatized individuals into the situation that induced the trauma.

PTSD induced by trauma of subordinates has likely been experienced by others, either as described here, or as a mixed form induced also by personal trauma. This form of PTSD is likely an important workplace hazard for civilian and military war commanders. This occupational hazard may select for leaders who are callous or are inured to the effects of it.

11

Shakespeare

SHAKESPEARE. THE NAME ITSELF indicates unparalleled descriptions of virtually any facet of nature or the human endeavor:

> *To gild refined gold, to paint the lily,/To throw a perfume on the violet,/*
> *To smooth the ice, or add another hue/Unto the rainbow*
> (King John 4.2.12–14).

> *Life's but a walking shadow, a poor player/That struts and frets his*
> *hour upon the stage /And then is heard no more* (Macbeth 5.5).

Or, miraculously, Shakespeare combines the natural and human:

> *There is a tide in the affairs of men,/Which, taken at the flood,*
> *leads on to fortune; /Omitted, all the voyage of their life /Is bound*
> *in shallows and in miseries./On such a full sea are we now afloat;*
> */And we must take the current when it serves,/Or lose our ventures.*
> (Julius Caesar 4.3)

As we have already seen in Chapter 10, Shakespeare wrote a complete, comprehensive and most beautiful description of a DSM-5 diagnosis of PTSD more than four hundred years before the DSM-5 was published! So it should come as no surprise that we can learn about medicine while reading additional works by Shakespeare. Perhaps we can even learn all that was known at his time, and much not known until our time nearly half a millennium later. There are articles written about medicine in Shakespeare on topics from ophthalmology and neurology to colorectal surgery, dermatology, rheumatology, and general surgery (Casey, 1967; Cosman, 1998; Cotterill, 1972; Erhlich, 1967; Fogan, 1989; Zekman and Davis, 1969).

Of course, not only does Shakespeare seem omniscient about medicine in his time and prescient about medicine in ours, he also has the incomparable ability to describe these diseases and conditions. King Richard III is believed to be disfigured from a possible problem associated with premature birth. But who among us could have thought to put this into words as the Bard did? A link between cerebral palsy and respiratory distress in premature birth is still being debated:

> *Cheated of feature by dissembling nature,*
> *Deformed, unfinish'd, sent before my time*
> *Into this breathing world, scarce half made up,*
> *And that so lamely and unfashionable*
> *That dogs bark at me as I halt by them;*

Richard III (1.1.19–23)

If Shakespeare's panoramic and all encompassing look at medicine in his time[1] is not remarkable enough, his look into the future is something to behold.

William Harvey (1578–1657) first demonstrated how blood circulates in 1616—the year of Shakespeare's death. Yet, in *Julius Caesar* (1599) Act 2, Scene 1, Brutus and Portia have the following exchange:

BRUTUS
You are my true and honourable wife,
As dear to me as are the ruddy drops
That visit my sad heart

PORTIA
If this were true, then should I know this secret.

Blood that returns to the heart that has had its oxygen extracted by body tissues is darker than blood emanating from the heart. Shakespeare's "ruddy drops" returning to the heart may indicate that he somehow knew the "secret" of blood circulation before Harvey.

Of course we can find other DSM-5 diagnoses besides PTSD in Shakespeare. In Chapter 9, we discussed sleep apnea (from the Greek *a* [not] + *pne* [breath or breathing]). In this condition (which can be associated with increased incidence of hypertension, heart disease, and potentially mortality), sufferers (most often obese individuals) have multiple episodes at night, while sleeping, where they literally stop breathing for some number of seconds. As a result, patients can suffer from daytime sleepiness (somnolence), and even decreased breathing (hypoventilation) during the day while awake. It is typically thought that Dickens was the first to describe sleep apnea in his novel the *Pickwick Papers*—decades before physicians diagnosed it. Yet, as Jack J. Adler pointed out in the *New England Journal of Medicine* more than 30 years ago (Adler, 1983), in *Henry IV* Shakespeare showed us his appreciation of the syndrome two and a half centuries earlier than Dickens! Shakespeare brilliantly captures this syndrome in just two lines:

> Peto
> *Falstaff! Fast asleep behind the arras, and snorting like a horse.*

> Prince
> *Hark, how hard he fetches breath. Search his pockets.*

> Henry IV (2.4.470–473)

In *Macbeth* we are introduced not only to psychiatric disease, but also to the field of psychiatry itself, even though the creation of the discipline lay centuries in the future. Act V, Scene 1 begins as the physic (doctor) and Lady Macbeth's Lady-in-Waiting wait to observe her sleepwalking and talking. It's the third night the two have been at the stakeout and, after the doctor's first comment you can feel him want to add the parenthetical that today's physicians would as well, "and I don't get reimbursed by the insurance company if the patient is a no-show!" The ever-observant physician notes that the patient's eyes are open—consistent with being awake—but Lady Macbeth's Lady completes the diagnosis noting that "their sense is shut." The doctor is careful to take notes for future reference. As occurs in modern medicine, after some observations the doctor feels the case is beyond his scope of practice and needs to refer to a specialist. By the time Lady Macbeth is finished with her sleepwalking activities the doctor is so amazed by what he has seen he thinks that indeed a higher power itself is needed to treat the patient.

> *SCENE I. Dunsinane. Ante-room in the castle.*

> *Enter a Doctor of Physic and a Waiting-Gentlewoman*

> Doctor
> *I have two nights watched with you, but can perceive*
> *no truth in your report. When was it she last walked?*

> Gentlewoman
> *Since his majesty went into the field, I have seen*
> *her rise from her bed, throw her night-gown upon*
> *her, unlock her closet, take forth paper, fold it,*
> *write upon't, read it, afterwards seal it, and again*
> *return to bed; yet all this while in a most fast sleep.*

Doctor
*A great perturbation in nature, to receive at once
the benefit of sleep, and do the effects of
watching! In this slumbery agitation, besides her
walking and other actual performances, what, at any
time, have you heard her say?*

Gentlewoman
That, sir, which I will not report after her.

Doctor
You may to me: and 'tis most meet you should.

Gentlewoman
*Neither to you nor any one; having no witness to
confirm my speech.*

Enter LADY MACBETH, with a taper

*Lo you, here she comes! This is her very guise;
and, upon my life, fast asleep. Observe her; stand close.*

Doctor
How came she by that light?

Gentlewoman
*Why, it stood by her: she has light by her
continually; 'tis her command.*

Doctor
You see, her eyes are open.

Gentlewoman
Ay, but their sense is shut.

Doctor
What is it she does now? Look, how she rubs her hands.

Gentlewoman
*It is an accustomed action with her, to seem thus
washing her hands: I have known her continue in
this a quarter of an hour.*

LADY MACBETH
Yet here's a spot.

Doctor
*Hark! she speaks: I will set down what comes from
her, to satisfy my remembrance the more strongly.*

LADY MACBETH
*Out, damned spot! out, I say!—One: two: why,
then, 'tis time to do't.—Hell is murky!—Fie, my
lord, fie! a soldier, and afeard? What need we
fear who knows it, when none can call our power to
account?—Yet who would have thought the old man
to have had so much blood in him.*

Doctor
Do you mark that?

LADY MACBETH
*The thane of Fife had a wife: where is she now?—
What, will these hands ne'er be clean?—No more o'
that, my lord, no more o' that: you mar all with
this starting.*

Doctor
Go to, go to; you have known what you should not.

Gentlewoman
*She has spoke what she should not, I am sure of
that: heaven knows what she has known.*

LADY MACBETH
*Here's the smell of the blood still: all the
perfumes of Arabia will not sweeten this little
hand. Oh, oh, oh!*

Doctor
What a sigh is there! The heart is sorely charged.

Gentlewoman
*I would not have such a heart in my bosom for the
dignity of the whole body.*

Doctor
Well, well, well, —

Gentlewoman
Pray God it be, sir.

Doctor
This disease is beyond my practise: yet I have known those which have walked in their sleep who have died holily in their beds.

LADY MACBETH
Wash your hands, put on your nightgown; look not so pale.—I tell you yet again, Banquo's buried; he cannot come out on's grave.

Doctor
Even so?

LADY MACBETH
To bed, to bed! there's knocking at the gate: come, come, come, come, give me your hand. What's done cannot be undone.—To bed, to bed, to bed!

Exit

Doctor
Will she go now to bed?

Gentlewoman
Directly.

Doctor
Foul whisperings are abroad: unnatural deeds
Do breed unnatural troubles: infected minds
To their deaf pillows will discharge their secrets:
More needs she the divine than the physician.
God, God forgive us all! Look after her;
Remove from her the means of all annoyance,
And still keep eyes upon her. So, good night:
My mind she has mated, and amazed my sight.
I think, but dare not speak.

Gentlewoman
Good night, good doctor.

Exeunt

Macbeth (5.1.1–80)

Beyond the medical descriptions and plot driving there is another interesting aspect of this scene. The doctor and lady-in-waiting are watching, as it were, a "performance" by Lady Macbeth. The scene is a play-within-a-play! Further, we are watching the whole thing: not only do we watch Lady Macbeth, and the doctor, and the lady-in-waiting, but, even more interesting for possible neuroscience and artistic study, we watch the doctor and lady-in-waiting *watching* Lady Macbeth![2]

In a most ingenious paper, Harrison Pope and colleagues (Pope et al., 2007) used a web-based challenge to complement their own investigations into looking for verifiable cases of **repressed memories**. Pope and colleagues have long challenged if there is such as thing as repressed memories at all. To qualify, a memory must be of an event occurring in an adult or older child—so that their brain is mature enough to form memories—that is forgotten for at least a year, and then remembered. In their paper Pope et al. noted that they had not found any verifiable examples of repressed memories in real people, and that, perhaps most interestingly, repressed memories appear to have arisen as a literary notion in the late 18th century. Indeed, neither Pope et al. nor any of the people who had responded to their challenge could find examples previous to this time.

When I read about their challenge, I thought back to a quick conversation that Professor Ramachandran and I had some years earlier. From time to time we discussed Shakespeare, and Rama would often quote his favorite passages (indeed, had science not been his calling, I think he would have made quite a good Shakespearean actor). One passage he quoted was from *Macbeth* Act 5, Scene 3. Rama knew about my interest in the history of medicine and literature and he said he thought that the passage presaged Freudian methods of psychoanalysis. He added that he had been alerted to the passage by his brother, V. S. Ravi, a policeman who is an academic "civilian"—neither professor nor physician—and a great lover of Shakespeare. When reading about the Pope challenge, I realized that not only did the passage Rama quoted predate Freud by centuries, but it discussed the topic of repressed memories. In Shakespeare's wonderful ambiguity, the passage leaves open the question of whether repressed memories exist. Also, unbelievably (though when it comes to the Bard perhaps this word should not be used), Shakespeare presages the modern controversy in the academic, medical, and lay public about repressed memories (Altschuler, Ramachandran, and Ravi, 2007).

MACBETH
How does your patient, doctor?

Doctor
Not so sick, my lord,
As she is troubled with thick coming fancies,
That keep her from her rest.

MACBETH
Cure her of that.
Canst thou not minister to a mind diseased,
Pluck from the memory a rooted sorrow,
Raze out the written troubles of the brain
And with some sweet oblivious antidote
Cleanse the stuff'd bosom of that perilous stuff
Which weighs upon the heart?

Doctor
Therein the patient
Must minister to himself[3]

Macbeth (5.3.3 7–41)

Is it possible to pick out a "most remarkable" medical occurrence in Shakespeare? There are so many remarkable quotes such as those discussed here. The portrayal of Sir Andrew Aguecheek in *Twelfth Night* not only stands out for its combination of pathophysiologic, neuropsychiatric, and even biochemical correctness, three and a half centuries ahead of its time, but also for its subtle—yet incisive—description of the medical problem and its impact on the character's persona. However, though the disease Shakespeare describes is not a DSM diagnosis, it brilliantly illustrates and illuminates the border and ambiguity of neurologic disease causing psychiatric symptoms—an instance of the dichotomies Shakespeare so often and effortlessly traffics in.

Sir Andrew was always thought by playgoers and scholars to be somewhat "slow." Sir Andrew himself recognizes this: (Act 1, Scene 3) "I am a fellow o' the strangest mind i' the/world," and (Act 2, Scene 5) "for many do call me fool."

But what, if anything in particular, was not fully appreciated until an article by British gastroenterologist William Summerskill in the *Lancet* in 1955 (Summerskill, 1955)? Summerskill points out that Sir Andrew is not retarded and had no congenital or other developmental problems since, as noted by Sir Toby Belch in Act 1, Scene 3, [Sir Andrew] plays o' the viol de gamboys, and speaks/three or four languages word for word without/the book and hath all the good gifts of Nature.

Then where and what is the problem? One clue comes from Maria's reproach to Sir Toby that Sir Andrew (Act 1, Scene 3) is "drunk nightly in your company." Today excess alcohol is known to cause liver cirrhosis. Shakespeare is on to this (Act 3, Scene 2) "For Andrew, if he were opened, and you/find so much blood in his liver as will/clog the foot of a flea, I'll eat the rest/of the anatomy."

Here is the genius. It was becoming known in the 1950s—though the full details are still not completely understood—that when high protein meals are eaten by individuals with significant liver cirrhosis, the liver is not able to fully process the nitrogen-containing chemical groups from the protein, and excess ammonia circulates in the body. Upon reaching the brain, the excess amonia plays a part in changing the individual's mental status, a condition called **hepatic encephalopathy**. (Today patients with cirrhotic liver disease often end up hospitalized after eating a high-protein fast food meal.) Sir Andrew and the Bard said it best (Act 1, Scene 3):

> *Methinks sometimes I have no more wit than*
> *a Christian or an ordinary man has; but I*
> *am a great eater of beef, and I believe that*
> *does harm to my wit.*

12

The Incredible Edgar Allan Poe

EDGAR ALLAN POE (1809–1849) was one of the greatest of all American writers and one of the first to emerge from the shadow of British dominance of English. He was a master of prose, poetry, and literary criticism, and a pioneer of the detective and horror story. But Poe's genius was not confined to the literary realm or even the humanities. Indeed, in his 1848 prose poem, "Eureka," Poe was the first to resolve Olbers' paradox (why the sky is dark at night) of cosmology and astrophysics. There are drawbacks to genius, however. Poe was also one of the most troubled and tragic of all American writers: he spent most of his life wracked by alcohol, monetary problems, and other indignities that left him dead at a young age.

When we look at Poe through a medical lens, we see that he was a remarkably innovative, accurate, and deep thinker. Consider the story of Phineas Gage—the railroad foreman whose skull and frontal lobe were impaled by a meter-long iron spike—which occurred in 1848 (Harlow, 1848). Gage remarkably not only survived, but after a period of recovery, he was able to walk, move his hands, and speak normally, and his cognition appeared not to have been grossly affected. While brain functions such as movement and cognition were not affected by the injury, Gage's personality was permanently changed: it was so negatively affected that his friends said that he was "no longer Gage." After the accident he never returned to his prior occupation. Amazingly, this syndrome that Gage suffered from, frontal lobe damage causing personality disorder (Table 12.1), unknown to the medical and science world until Gage's freak accident in 1848, was described by Poe in 1840 (Altschuler, 2004; Altschuler and Augenstein, 2012)!

In Poe's story *Peter Pendulum, The Business Man* (published in *Burton's Gentleman's Magazine*; February, 1840; 6: 897–899) the protagonist of the

TABLE 12.1 Symptoms of Frontal Lobe Syndrome
Depending on the location and extent of injury symptoms can include:
Social and behavior changes
Exacerbation of pre-existing behavioral traits such as disorderliness, suspiciousness, argumentativeness, disruptiveness, and anxiousness
Apathy, loss of interest in social interactions, lack of concern for consequences of behavior
Lewdness, loss of social graces, inattention to personal hygiene and appearance
Boisterousness, intrusiveness, increased volume of speech, excessive profanity
Increased risk taking including excessive alcohol and illegal drug use, gluttony and indiscriminate food selection
Impulsivity and distractibility
Affective changes
Apathy, indifference
Lability of affect, irritability, manic states
Poor behavioral control, fits of rage and violent behavior
Intellectual changes
Reduced capacity for language, symbols and logic
Reduced ability to use mathematics or process information, reduced reasoning ability
Diminished ability to focus or concentrate

Source: After Mackinnon and Yudofsky, 1986; Yudofsky and Silver, 1987.

story interestingly describes himself from the outset: "I am a business-man. I am a methodical man. Method is the thing, after all. But there are no people I more heartily despise than your eccentric fools who prate about method without understanding it; attending strictly to its letter, and violating its spirit." He credits his sense of order with a formative child-hood accident: "A good-hearted old Irish nurse (whom I shall not forget in my will) took me up one day by the heels, when I was making more noise than was necessary, and swinging me round two or three times . . . and then knocked my head into a cocked hat against the bedpost. This, I say, decided my fate, and made my fortune. A bump arose at once on my sinciput [forehead], and turned out to be as pretty an organ of order as one shall see on a summer's day."

But this Businessman cannot even keep a job, lasting in most for a few months or less, typically quitting or being fired after a squabble with employers whom he feels do not appreciate his sense of order. The jobs are as flawed as the entrepreneur who perpetrates them; one job is in the

"Assault-and-Battery business," and he is jailed once for his enterprising actions—lamp-blacking a client's building. Aspects of the frontal-lobe syndrome suffered by the Businessman include his obsessive interest in and devotion to order, his flat affect, and poor functioning in society. Characteristics seen in patients with pediatric injuries (Poe was centuries ahead of his time in appreciating the pediatric frontal lobe syndrome [Anderson et al., 1999]) such as antisocial behavior—e.g., violent occupations and incarceration—and no insight into the thinking processes of others, are also noted.

In 1845 Poe published another version of the story named simply *The Business Man* (*Broadway Journal* 1845; August, 2 2: 49–52), five paragraphs longer and including four more jobs the man had and lost, than in the original version. Why did Poe add to the story? In medicine, when a doctor is trying to diagnosis a complex case, the old dictum is "repeat the history and physical examination." Perhaps this is what Poe was doing with the 1845 revised version: the protagonist's history is expanded on, and the additional jobs that are lost are indeed confirmatory and consistent with the diagnosis of frontal lobe syndrome.

How could Poe have known about frontal lobe syndrome, a disorder not appreciated by physicians and scientists until the dramatic event of Gage's, years after Poe published the Businessman stories? Further, Poe also seems to understand the severity of the syndrome when it starts in childhood. Presumably, Poe must have used his keen observational and deductive powers to link a frontal lobe injury to a change in behavior in someone he knew from childhood. The titular Businessman mentions in his diatribe that, "In biography the truth is everything—and in autobiography, especially so. . ." But the question of who is the inspiration for the brain-injured nuisance of Poe's story is destined to remain buried with Poe. Like all great art, it also leaves us with nuances and questions to ponder evermore. Poe's diagnostic coup remains; his 1840 piece is the earliest, and still one of the finest and most gripping descriptions of frontal lobe syndrome in print.

Today, Poe's story retains not only great interest—it's a great read—but it's also important and useful for our purposes of examining the earliest case studies of mental illness. Indeed, traumatic brain injury is the number one cause of death and disability worldwide, with millions of cases annually. Around ten percent of these cases are moderate or severe, with ninety percent being mild and quite possibly presenting with symptoms of frontal lobe damage, a common site of damage in traumatic brain injury, or symptoms of damage to other brain areas. Symptoms and signs of neurologic disease from brain damage and other causes can be far more insidious and harder to diagnose than those of psychiatric disease. Thus, lessons from Poe's story can be useful. Curiously, in many cases we have very good or even excellent medicines, therapies, and other means to treat psychiatric diseases such as depression and schizophrenia; however, there are often no treatments for symptoms of neurologic disease.

There is more neuroscience and medicine in Poe: Poe's 1839 story, *William Wilson,* contains a particularly vivid depiction of heautoscopy (seeing oneself at a distance) (Brugger et al., 1994). Synesthesia is a neurologic phenomenon experienced by 1–2 percent of the population in which the experience of one sensation automatically stimulates that of another. For example, the most common form of synesthesia is grapheme-color synesthesia, whereby the letter "A" might always be seen in red, or the number "7" in blue. Other individuals report associating certain shapes to specific tastes. Peter Brugger from the Department of Neurology at University Hospital in Zurich found (Knoch et al., 2005) the earliest known example of bidirectional synesthesia in Poe's *Marginalia Part I* (*Democratic Review,* November 1844, pp. 484–494, p. 490): "The orange ray of the spectrum and the buzz of the gnat (which never rises above the second A), affect me with nearly similar sensations. In hearing the gnat, I perceive the color. In perceiving the color, I seem to hear the gnat." Curiously, Poe's originality may be most outstanding with respect to the medical and scientific[1].

Interesting and particularly haunting is Poe's early description not of a disease, but of a medical procedure—that of obtaining informed consent (Altschuler, 2003). These days, before performing any invasive procedure such as an operation, injection, or even certain diagnostic tests that might have risks of side effects associated with them—to get a biopsy, for example—physicians must obtain informed consent. Informed consent informs patients about the risks and benefits of the procedure and then, if the patient has the capability to do so, the patient decides whether or not they want the operation or other medical intervention. (This is true in research studies as well; people must be informed of the risks and benefits involved in participating in a study before agreeing to participate.)

Poe's 1845 story, *The Facts in the Case of M. Valdemar,* is a gripping narrative. A certain P, the narrator and protagonist of the story, starts the story by discussing research on Mesmerism, or hypnotism: "My attention, for the last three years, had been repeatedly drawn to the subject of Mesmerism; and, about nine months ago it occurred to me, quite suddenly, that in the series of experiments made hitherto, there had been a very remarkable and most unaccountable omission: no person had as yet been mesmerized in *articulo mortis* [at the point of death]. It remained to be seen, first, whether, in such condition, there existed in the patient any susceptibility to the magnetic influence; secondly, whether, if any existed, it was impaired or increased by the condition; thirdly, to what extent, or for how long a period, the encroachments of Death might be arrested by the process. There were other points to be ascertained, but these most excited my curiosity—the last in especial, from the immensely important character of its consequences."

P then searches for an appropriate subject and finds one in his friend, Monsieur Ernest Valdemar, whose death within one day (by Sunday morning) from pulmonary tuberculosis and a possible aortic aneurysm, had been certifiably predicted by two doctors. At 7:55 on Saturday night, in the presence of Mr. L (a medical student and note-taker, also serving the function of what today would be considered a witness), P took hold of Valdemar's hand and "begged him to state, as distinctly as he could, to Mr. L whether he (M. Valdemar) was entirely willing that I should make the experiment of mesmerizing him in his then condition. He replied feebly, yet quite audibly, 'Yes, I wish to be mesmerized'." The experiment proceeded.

Valdemar is kept in this twilit, dead but aware state for seven months. He has no pulse and is not breathing, but hypnotically responds to the physician's questions. Throughout the narrative, it's clear that Poe avidly studied medical texts for his authoritative medical voice in the story. That voice especially rings true when he comes to the supernatural twist at the ending: as Valdemar finally convinces the mesmerist to make a choice between life and death, his body instantly and graphically begins to decay to "detestable putrescence" in front of the narrator's eyes.

Death is ever present in Poe's writings. There has been some study on the cause of Poe's own death. It has long been assumed that he died of causes related to alcoholism, but there have been recent debates. A historical clinical pathological group at the University of Maryland suggested that Poe may have died of rabies (Benitez, 1996). Near the time of Poe's death, symptoms such as fear of drinking water (hydrophobia) and looking at himself in a mirror were reported. These symptoms can accompany an infection with rabies as potential evidence for this diagnosis. Perhaps it is not surprising, and maybe it's even fitting, that there remains some mystery surrounding Poe's death.

13

Heracles and Homer

ARE THERE LITERARY CHARACTERS, other than Samson
(see Chapter 1), who had ASPD? Perhaps the most significant issue
when diagnosing ASPD is not having complete information about the
patient. So this search through the literary past is not as simple as it might
seem at first.

Before we get to Heracles and Homer, let's consider a few other characters, beginning with the biblical character, Cain. True, Cain killed his
brother Abel and then lied to God when asked if had committed the
crime. While Cain's misdeed was a horrible act, and one committed in the
context of family/social pathology, there is no further evidence that Cain
committed other misdeeds or antisocial acts, so it would be irresponsible
to diagnose Cain with ASPD.

What about the Greek mythology character, Achilles? Certainly he
killed many people in battle, and *The Iliad* documents cruelties committed by Achilles, but also by many others. As United States Army Union
Major General William T. Sherman commented, "war is hell." Did Achilles' actions stand out from this context as particularly antisocial? I believe
not. Indeed, the returning of Hector's body to his father Priam, King of
Troy by Achilles is the antithesis of an antisocial act; rather, it's an act of
compassion.

What about Heracles, another character from Greek mythology? Here
I believe that the diagnosis does fit, but it takes a great effort to make it
fit due to limited information. Diagnosing Heracles with ASPD high-
lights the importance of having enough information upon which to base
the diagnosis. Where does our information about Heracles come from?
Unfortunately, unlike the biblical story of Samson there is not one old,
long coherent text. The earliest literary mentions of Heracles can be found
in Homer's *The Iliad* and *The Odyssey*. However, it is clear from reading

Homer that the Heracles stories, such as those of *Heracles 12 Labors*, date from some time—not fully specified—before the time of the writing (if not the occurrence) of the events described[1] in *The Iliad* and *The Odyssey*. Another potential source for older material on Heracles would be fine art. However, I am not aware of any piece that depicts Heracles and that is reliably dated before the Homeric myths. So our oldest evidence about Heracles is "Homer's Heracles," or at least Homer's transcription of older known stories. Conversely, the most substantial and longest ancient text on Heracles comes from the Latin poet Ovid (43 BC–17 AD) in Book 9 of his *Metamorphoses*. So we want to consider Ovid's Heracles as well.

Book 5, lines 648–651 of *The Iliad* describe how, in a past time, Heracles destroyed Troy after he was treated poorly by the Trojan King Laomedon (father of the Trojan King Priam of Homeric fame). Apparently, Heracles was provoked, but his response—destroying a city—seems a bit extreme. Indeed, the thoroughness of the destruction is emphasized in Book 14, line 251.

Heracles is featured in two places in *The Odyssey*. In Book 11, Odysseus visits Hades to get advice, counsel, and information from various "shades" and "spirits" there. He encounters Heracles near the very end of the book (lines 599–628). Heracles does not act in a particularly antisocial way in this Book, but Homer notes that the other spirits were frightened of Heracles, who was carrying a bow and arrow. Odysseus' hackles were raised as well. At the very least this shows that Heracles was a frightening and potentially violent individual, though Heracles commiserates with Odysseus, comparing Odysseus' wanderings to his own labors.

In Book 21 (lines 24–29), we find the strongest evidence that Heracles may have had ASPD. Here he kills Iphitos in order to steal and keep Iphitos' horses. There is no sign that Heracles shows any remorse for his act. Today, in many jurisdictions, this would carry a sentence of death because, while committing murder, Heracles also committed another felony—robbery. Recall that Samson committed this same heinous dual crime.

Thus, in Homer, we see that Heracles certainly meets the ASPD criteria for aggressiveness, as he is repeatedly involved in fights and physical acts of violence. Heracles, too, can show lack of remorse. At times he also shows disregard for the safety of others.

Another very significant literary source of information about Heracles was written at least 8 centuries after Homer by the great Roman poet, Publius Ovidius Naso—best known as Ovid—in Book 9 of his masterwork, *Metamorphoses*. Ovid talks mostly about Heracles' acts of great strength, such as killing two snakes with his bare hands that tried to kill him while he was still a baby in his cradle, to Heracles' twelve great labors as an adult. Though these are certainly violent acts, often Heracles is defending himself from various mortal threats, so I do not see this text as particularly valuable in diagnosing Heracles with ASPD. Also, while Ovid is a master raconteur, there is a distance from any possible real model in Ovid, contrasting with a certain sense of proximity that one feels exists between Heracles and Homer—due to Homer's great story-telling and also the time (and culture) of Homer seeming closer to the age of Heracles than Ovid's work.

Another ingenious medical point about Heracles was made by Branimir Čatipović in a short letter (Čatipović, 2004) in the *New England Journal of Medicine*. A protein called myostatin was found some years previously, which, when mutated, causes increased muscle mass. This mutation was found first in mice, then in cattle, and then in a case report (Schuelke, et al., 2004) of a human child that Čatipović commented on. "Myo" is the Greek word for muscle and "statin" is the Latin word for stop; this protein puts the brakes on muscle growth, lest it get too big and bulky for the rest of the body to support. The mice, cows, and the child had much greater muscle bulk than is considered within normal range. For example, the child had substantial muscle bulk observable at birth, and at age 4.5 years could hold two 3kg weights out horizontally. Čatipović made the ingenious suggestion that this child may not have been the first case of myostatin deficiency in humans, but that Heracles was! Čatipović noted Heracles' great strength from birth as evidenced by his killing of a snake with each hand while an infant. Also, as Čatipović pointed out, Heracles' strength was never attributed to an exercise or dietary regimen. One wonders if there could have been a real person who had myostatin deficiency that Heracles was modeled after.

I noticed an interesting medical footnote about Heracles some years ago during an exhibit, *The Golden Deer of Eurasia: Scythian and Sarmatian Treasures from the Russian Steppes*, at the Metropolitan Museum of Art (Alt-schuler, 2001; Aruz et al., 2000). This exhibit had remarkable pieces from the Russian Steppes. One particular piece, a vessel or a cup, featured a relief frieze that showed a timeless exemplar of medical compassion and care: One man tending the wounds of another. Additional figures on the cup told the story of the founding myth of Scythia as recounted in Book 4.8–10 of Herodatus' *Histories*: Heracles had been to the land of Scythia where a strange maiden/serpent consort of his bore him three children. He told the mother-to-be that when the children grew older to have them each try to string a bow that Heracles left behind. The one who did would be King. Neither of the two older brothers, Agathyrsus or Gelonus, could string the bow. (The injuries they sustained while trying are shown on the vessel.) But the youngest son, Scythes, could string the bow, and the kingdom was thus founded.

This footnote turns out to have a footnote of its own. Using the ability to string a bow as a test of kingship is not confined to Scythes and the Scythian founding myth. Homer uses it in Book 21 of *The Odyssey*! Potential suitors for Odysseus' wife Penelope tried to string Odysseus' bow. (Of course, only Odysseus in disguise could do so.) Cleary there is a Freudian component to the task, which could have led to independent discovery and use of this task by the authors of the Scythian founding myth and Homer in *The Odyssey*. However, I find it more likely that the author of one myth borrowed the idea from the other. Or might somehow the same author have composed both stories?

14

The Brain That Kills the Heart
Death in a James Joyce Story

ONE DAY, EARLY IN MY JUNIOR YEAR of high school, Mr. Watras, the fearsome (but beloved) band director/conductor and Assistant Principal, asked a couple of us in the orchestra if we wanted to go to a chamber music concert that night at Lincoln Center. Mr. Watras didn't usually talk to orchestra members about orchestra matters per se—and this was clearly an "orchestra type" concert, not a band concert. Mr. Watras wasn't the kind of person you say "no" to, so of course we accepted the tickets. He was a bit inscrutable, and I still can't decide whether he thought that we specifically should go to the concert or that the Board of Education wanted students attending, and Mr. Watras was going to make sure Stuyvesant High School sent the most students.

The concert featured pieces by Haydn and Faure, but more curious were three early unpublished songs for mezzo-soprano and piano by Viennese composer Alban Berg (1885–1935), that were having their American debut that night by Frederica von Stade and pianist Richard Goode. The scores for the pieces came from the Robert O. Lehman collection of music manuscripts at the Morgan Library (the score of one piece was printed in the program and I still regret not keeping that program).

Berg was the finest student of the composer and music theorist Arnold Schoenberg (1874–1951), the founder of the so-called second "Viennese school of composing" (the first Viennese school is a bit of a mythical entity but includes Haydn, Mozart, Beethoven, and Schubert). Berg had done quite a lot of composing—mostly piano music and songs—before coming under Schoenberg's tutelage. Schoenberg taught Berg his so-called "serialist" or 12-tone style, in which a piece was based not on a beautiful sounding melody as in the history of music until the twentieth century, but on an arrangement of all twelve notes of the scale (with no repetitions)—the so-called "tone row." Berg's lyricism allowed him to not only far surpass his teacher, but even make 12-tone music sound beautiful.

But the song set that night was Berg pre-Schoenberg and was truly incredible. It was romantic, like a set of Brahms songs—yet "post-Brahms" with daring and striking harmonies that were "twentieth century" without being abstract or pedantic. Of course, Berg's natural lyricism brought the pieces to vibrant life. When listening I felt like I was hearing the answer to the "question" of what the nineteenth century would be like if extended into the twentieth century.

Many (many) years later, I was glancing at James Joyce's (1882–1941) collection of short stories, *Dubliners,* and the story titled "A Painful Case" caught my eye. Though *Dubliners* was not published until 1914, most of the stories from the collection, including "A Painful Case," were written in 1905, long before Joyce wrote the more abstract and difficult novels *Ulysses* (1918–1920) and *Finnegan's Wake* (1939). "The Painful Case" and the other stories do not disappoint (Altschuler, 2008) and are worthy of nineteenth century masters such as Poe, Dickens, and Stevenson, but like Berg's songs, convey a feeling of being "twentieth century," not only in regards to the era and characters, but also because of certain aspects of writing style, such as blending narrative and textual criticism. Miraculously, "Painful Case" also provides us with a glimpse into the heart and mind nearly a century before the now all-prevalent CT ("cat") scans, MRI, and other testing and imaging now commonly used to diagnose internal and mental disease and disorder. Joyce's "case" juxtaposes and combines a DSM disorder—alcohol abuse disorder—with a neurologic disorder, resulting in a mysterious and powerful general medical effect that is reminiscent of many of the great works we have discussed.

The plot of "A Painful Case" revolves around the story behind the newspaper headline "Death of a Lady at Sydney Parade: A Painful Case." The Deputy Coroner (at the City of Dublin hospital) was investigating the death of 43-year-old Mrs. Emily Sinico the previous evening. Witnesses testified that at ten in the evening, as the slow train was pulling out of Sydney Parade Station, Mrs. Sinico attempted to cross the train line and was caught by the buffer of the engine and fell to the ground before bystanders could stop her. Both the police sergeant and constable testified that Mrs. Sinico was dead upon their arrival at the station. Dr. Halpin, an assistant house surgeon at the City of Dublin Hospital, testified that Mrs. Sinico had fractured two lower ribs, sustained a severe contusion to the right shoulder, and an injury to the right side of the head, but that "the injuries were not sufficient to have caused death in a normal person. Death, in his opinion, was probably due to shock and sudden failure of the heart's action." Mrs. Sinico was not known to have had any medical problems. Her daughter noted for two years prior to her death that Mrs. Sinico had been in the nightly habit of going out and buying spirits (alcohol). The story reveals that this two-year period began with the break-up of an intense, but platonic, relationship between Mrs. Sinico and one Mr. James Duffy, the story's protagonist.

Joyce, with the steady hand of the master artist, was calculating in his details here. Mrs. Sinico's death is not simply "pure fiction." In the medical world today it is well-known that brain contusion or hemorrhage (e.g., from spontaneous aneurysm rupture or blunt trauma), can cause sudden cardiopulmonary arrest (Estanol and Marin, 1975; Tabaaa et al., 1987). Case reports suggest that individuals with a history of alcohol abuse may be particularly susceptible to this (Milovanovic and DiMaio, 1999). A number of possible mechanisms by which brain contusion can lead to cardiopulmonary arrest have been identified such as cardiac arrhythmias secondary to a massive release of catecholamines (i.e., epinephrine and related molecules) and respiratory arrest secondary to compression of respiratory centers in the brain. Interestingly, in 1889, physician and electrophysiologist John MacWilliam (MacWilliam, 1889) was remarkably prescient in suggesting that a brain hemorrhage could cause cardiac fibrillation, an idea not developed until nearly a century later by electrocardiography. Joyce's story seems to be the first detailed human "case report" of the brain contusion/sudden cardiopulmonary arrest syndrome. Indeed, the fact that Joyce has two police officers—the sergeant and the constable—testify that the lady was dead before they arrived at the station, seems to indicate that Joyce wants to emphasize and let us know that he knows, the sudden nature of the death from this condition. He was playing literary doctor, and doing it quite ahead of his time.

It is well known that from a relatively early age Joyce drank heavily. Thus, issues in "A Painful Case" relating to alcohol probably derived from the author's personal knowledge and motivation. We have seen the deleterious effects of alcohol and substance abuse in Stevenson and Gogol. It is not readily apparent how Joyce might have known about the adverse effects that brain injury might have on the heart—whether Joyce was somehow aware of the work and theories of MacWilliam or others on the topic or not. We have seen this kind of combination of neurologic and medical problem in the Bard. There is enough specificity and clarity in the description of the medical case in this story, though not without some ambiguity, to propose that Joyce was suggesting a pathophysiologic role of brain injury in the cause of Mrs. Sinico's death by cardiopulmonary arrest, rather than a non-specific and metaphorical connection between the brain and the heart. Was he writing about his own drinking and its destructive powers? Was he commenting, perhaps metaphorically, that a blunt trauma from a metaphorical engine of technology and modernity had caused a literal heartbreak in the disappointed, down-and-out woman? One can wonder forever: Joyce's specificity and clarity, coupled with just enough ambiguity in the medical case description, and all other aspects of the story gives "A Painful Case" it's wonderful immortality.

A couple of years ago I found what I believe is an interesting footnote to "A Painful Case." Joyce was a great enthusiast of astronomy. Indeed, Chapter 17 of *Ulysses* has fifty passages of astronomical interest and the rest of the book includes references to a solar eclipse, the phases of the moon, constellations, and the supernova of 1572 (Olson 2014). In one section of Chapter 17, Bloom and Dedalus see a meteor and note that they also hear the "sound of the peal of the hour of the night by the chime of the bells in the church of Saint George … Heigho, heigho, Heigho, heigho." This pattern of bells is that of Westminster Chimes of the half-hour. Physics professor Donald Olson and English professor Margaret Olson, a husband and wife team from Texas State University in San Marcos, used astronomical and other sleuthing to figure out (Olson and Olson, 2004) that bells were tolling at 1:30 a.m. and that Joyce's meteor appeared near the bright stars of Lyra. The Lyrid meteor shower was first described by astronomer Stand Dvorak in 1966 (Dvorak, 1966). Thus, like Poe, Joyce made original contributions to both the medical and astronomical literature.

15

Using the DSM-5

WE HAVE SEEN MANY EXAMPLES of DSM-5-specific diagnoses in literature. But, how does one go about using the DSM-5 in practice?

The first thing to do when considering DSM-5 diagnoses in a patient is to take a thorough history and conduct a physical examination. Then, based on the history and physical exam, the patient may need some labs, imaging, or other tests. When these tests are complete, and other medical issues are ruled out or discovered, you are probably ready to examine the patient for a DSM-5 diagnosis. The list of categories of diagnoses can be found at https://www.psychiatry.org/psychiatrists/practice/dsm.

The next step is to assess—given the patient's history, physical exam, tests, and further questioning—if the patient fits criteria for a given diagnosis. In the literary cases and characters we examined here, patients often have a single diagnosis—a useful literary approach—yet patients in the clinic may have more than one diagnosis. A good DSM-5 diagnosis lists all applicable diagnoses.

The DSM-5 encourages the practitioner to consider general medical issues that may be contributing to or exacerbating a patient's psychiatric disease. The DSM-5 also encourages the practitioner to consider social, economic, workplace, family, and other factors that may be stressors on the patient, and also to consider the patient's overall functioning in social, work, and educational settings. The DSM-5 encourages the clinician to assess the severity of a patient's disease for each diagnosis. For some diagnoses, e.g., mood disorders, schizophrenia, and substance-related disorders, the DSM-5 includes specific diagnosis modifiers that can be attached to the diagnosis. The clinician is advised to consider whether a diagnosis is present in a given patient in mild, moderate, severe, or extreme form.

Epilogue

A License to Make Literary Diagnoses

IN THIS BOOK WE HAVE SEEN how examples from great literature can been most useful in learning how to use the DSM-5. The DSM-5 is just one tool in diagnosing a patient or research subject. Diagnosing a patient requires a thorough and careful medical and social history and physical examination. Also, with increasing experience one's diagnostic skills grow.

But it may be time to issue a license to diagnose literary characters. Remember our friend, the Nobel Prize winning physicist Richard Feynman from the Introduction, who spoke of "… the simplicity we typically associate with truth"? When trying to diagnose figures from great literature there can often be a simplicity not always present when trying to diagnose patients. This simplicity typically originates with the author who, when appropriate, builds it in to make a literary "case" clear: For example, Gogol made it a point to have Poprischin and Major Kovalyov at a key juncture exclaim that they do not drink. These proclamations are crucial exclusion criteria needed to "clear the deck" and permit consideration of other psychiatric diagnoses. Or at the key moment when his former boss sees Bartleby in jail, Melville has him note, "I know you, and I want nothing to say to you." And a bit later, "I know where I am," thus simplifying things by effectively excluding a thought disorder (schizophrenia) or delirium.

You are ready and credentialed to go forth and diagnose literary characters. When you find an interesting case, please let me know!

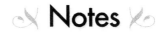

Notes

Introduction Notes

1. Number of the Insane and Idiotic, with brief Notices of the Lunatic Asylums in the United States. *American Journal of Insanity* 1844; 1: 78–88. (Articles in the early issues of the journals did not list authors.)

2. Interestingly, the second and longest article in the first issue of the journal was a study of insanity in history, literature and poetry! Insanity—illustrated by histories of distinguished men, and by the writings of poets and novelists. *American Journal of Insanity* 1844; 1: 9–46. I don't find any examples given in this article that meet DSM-5 criteria for insanity (schizophrenia) or any related diagnoses.

Chapter 2 Notes

1. I thank the staff at the UCSD bookstore for introducing me to Gogol's wonderful story. I also thank Suzy Conway (Harvard Medical School Countway Library) for helpful discussions; and Jonathan Saville (UCSD) for invaluable discussions and for confirming, by reading this story in Russian, that the diagnosis is not an artifact produced by translation.

Chapter 4 Notes

1. D.C.L. is a Doctor of Civil Laws; LL. D. is a Doctor of Laws—the highest law degree or an honorary degree; FRS is a Fellow of the Royal Society—the highest scientific honor.

2. Stevenson was desperately in need of money in October 1885 and was scrambling for a story that could lift his finances. The plot for *Jekyll and Hyde* appeared on the second night of particularly intense brain wracking. Stevenson wrote the first draft of *Jekyll and Hyde* in only three days, and then, as he was unsatisfied with this draft, burned it, and rewrote the novella in three more days. He wrote a very impressive 60,000 words in just six days. Was such output simply the product of economic necessity and desperation? Or, might Stevenson have written the

story in the midst of a manic episode? (It's thought that Handel wrote a significant part of his *Messiah,* including the *Hallelujah Chorus,* in two weeks during such an episode.) Alternatively, Myron Schultz suggested some decades ago (1971) that Stevenson's brisk writing was fueled by cocaine. Schultz speculated that Stevenson got the idea to use cocaine from his wife who was always looking for a new cure for Stevenson's chronic lung ailment and bleeding. Schultz mentions that an article appearing in the *Lancet* in September 1885 might have caught Fanny Stevenson's eye. I haven't been able to locate this article. However, cocaine was all the rage in the medical and popular press at that time as a wonder drug following the report in September 1884 by Viennese ophthalmologist Carl Koller about the stunning local anesthetic effects of cocaine on the eye.
3. The DSM-5 expanded the substance use disorder chapter to include an activity as a substance with potential for use disorder—gambling disorder. Reader's of Dostyevsky's *The Gambler* (1867) would not have found this new.

Chapter 5 Notes

1. The only significant change in the DSM-5 to criteria for major depressive disorder is removal of the so-called bereavement exclusion: In DSM-IV if an individual met criteria for an episode of major depression but this episode followed the death of a loved one and was confined to within two months of the death, then the diagnosis of major depression was automatically excluded. This exclusion was removed both because depression following the death of a loved one can last longer than two months, and also to recognize and appreciate the importance, significance, and at times severity of a veritable episode of major depression occurring (even a short time) following the passing of a loved one.

But the idea that a true major depressive episode can follow the death of a loved one is certainly not new. In fact, it dates practically back to the dawn of the history of medicine—to written texts that have a relation to medicine. Bermejo (Description d'une depression vieille de 3300 ans. *Revue Médicale de la Suisse Romande* 1998; 118: 509) discusses a letter addressed to Eneade—the court of the Gods beyond (M. Guilmont. Lettre à une épousé defunte. [Pap. Leiden 1, 37]). *ZÄS Zeitschrift für aegyptische Sprache und Altertumskunde* 1973; 99: 94–103) that was mentioned in a book by Dondelinger Edmund et Florence Delay (*Le Livre Sacré de L'Ancienne Égypte* [Phillippe Lebaud, Paris, 1987]) by a grieving widower whose wife died eight months earlier. The husband complains that he is bewitched by the Perfect Ghost of Ankh-Iri, his wife, whom he says does not leave him alone. The letter states that continuing for eight months since his wife's death he is not eating as usual and "his joy" is in a "painful state." The letter

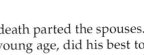

describes a happy, indeed idyllic, life before death parted the spouses. The husband notes that he got married at a young age, did his best to feed his wife and make her happy, never committed adultery, and when his wife was diagnosed with an incurable disease he called the chief physician. When his wife died, he provided the nicest clothes to bury her in and cried with the other members of the family. Given this righteous and conscientious behavior the husband is surprised his wife's ghost continues to torment him.

Chapter 8 Notes

TABLE 8.2 Diagnostic Criteria for Generalized Anxiety Disorder

A. Excessive anxiety and worry (apprehensive expectation), occurring more days than not for at least 6 months, about a number of events or activities (such as work or school performance).

B. The individual finds it difficult to control the worry.

C. The anxiety and worry are associated with three (or more) of the following six symptoms (with at least some symptoms having been present for more days than not for the past 6 months)[1]:

   1. Restlessness or feeling keyed up or on edge

   2. Being easily fatigued

   3. Difficulty concentrating or mind going blank

   4. Irritability

   5. Muscle tension

   6. Sleep disturbance (difficulty falling or staying asleep, or restless, unsatisfying sleep).

D. The anxiety, worry, or physical symptoms cause clinically significant distress or impairment in social, occupational, or other important areas of functioning.

E. The disturbance is not attributable to the physiological effects of a substance (e.g., a drug of abuse, a medication) or another medical condition (e.g., hyperthyroidism).

F. The disturbance is not better explained by another mental disorder (e.g., anxiety or worry about having panic attacks in panic disorder, negative evaluation in social anxiety disorder [social phobia], contamination or other obsessions in obsessive-compulsive disorder, separation from attachment figures in separation anxiety disorder, reminders of traumatic events in posttraumatic stress disorder, gaining weight in anorexia nervosa, physical complaints in somatic symptom disorder, perceived appearance flaws in body dysmorphic disorder, having a serious illness in illness anxiety disorder, or the content of delusional beliefs in schizophrenia or delusional disorder).

[1]Only one item is required in children.

(Reprinted with permission from the *Diagnostic and Statistical Manual of Mental Disorders, Fifth Edition,* © 2013. American Psychiatric Association.)

TABLE 8.3 ⟍ Diagnostic Criteria for Dysthymic Disorder

A. Depressed mood for most of the day, for more days than not, as indicated either by subjective account or observation by others, for at least 2 years. Note: In children and adolescents, mood can be irritable and duration must be at least 1 year.

B. Presence, while depressed, of two (or more) of the following:

    1. Poor appetite or overeating

    2. Insomnia or hypersomnia

    3. Low energy or fatigue

    4. Low self-esteem

    5. Poor concentration or difficulty making decisions

    6. Feelings of hopelessness

C. During the 2-year period (1 year for children or adolescents) of the disturbance, the person has never been without the symptoms in Criteria A and B for more than 2 months at a time.

D. No Major Depressive Episode has been present during the first 2 years of the disturbance (1 year for children and adolescents); i.e., the disturbance is not better accounted for by chronic Major Depressive Disorder, or Major Depressive Disorder, in partial remission.

    Note: There may have been a previous Major Depressive Episode provided there was a full remission (no significant signs or symptoms for 2 months) before development of the Dysthymic Disorder. In addition, after the initial 2 years (1 year in children or adolescents) of Dysthymic Disorder, there may be superimposed episodes of Major Depressive Disorder, in which case both diagnoses may be given when the criteria are met for a Major Depressive Episode.

E. There has never been a Manic Episode, a Mixed Episode, or a Hypomanic Episode, and criteria have never been met for Cyclothymic Disorder.

F. The disturbance does not occur exclusively during the course of a chronic Psychotic Disorder, such as Schizophrenia or Delusional Disorder.

G. The symptoms are not due to the direct physiological effects of a substance (e.g., a drug of abuse, a medication) or a general medical condition (e.g., hypothyroidism).

H. The symptoms cause clinically significant distress or impairment in social, occupational, or other important areas of functioning.

(Reprinted with permission from the *Diagnostic and Statistical Manual of Mental Disorders, Fifth Edition,* © 2013. American Psychiatric Association.)

TABLE 8.4 ⟍ Diagnostic Criteria for Obsessive-Compulsive Disorder

A. Presence of obsessions, compulsions, or both:

    Obsessions are defined by (1) and (2):

    1. Recurrent and persistent thoughts, urges, or images that are experienced, at some time during the disturbance, as intrusive and unwanted, and that in most individuals cause marked anxiety or distress.

TABLE 8.4 (continued)

2. The individual attempts to ignore or suppress such thoughts, urges, or images, or to neutralize them with some other thought or action (i.e., by performing a compulsion).

Compulsions are defined by (1) and (2):

1. Repetitive behaviors (e.g., hand washing, ordering, checking) or mental acts (e.g., praying, counting, repeating words silently) that the individual feels driven to perform in response to an obsession or according to rules that must be applied rigidly.

2. The behaviors or mental acts are aimed at preventing or reducing anxiety or distress, or preventing some dreaded event or situation; however, these behaviors or mental acts are not connected in a realistic way with what they are designed to neutralize or prevent, or are clearly excessive.

Note: Young children may not be able to articulate the aims of these behaviors or mental acts.

B. The obsessions or compulsions are time-consuming (e.g., take more than 1 hour per day) or cause clinically significant distress or impairment in social, occupational, or other important areas of functioning.

C. The obsessive-compulsive symptoms are not attributable to the physiological effects of a substance (e.g., a drug of abuse, a medication) or another medical condition.

D. The disturbance is not better explained by the symptoms of another mental disorder (e.g., excessive worries, as in generalized anxiety disorder; preoccupation with appearance, as in body dysmorphic disorder; difficulty discarding or parting with possessions, as in hoarding disorder; hair pulling, as in trichotillomania [hair-pulling disorder]; skin picking, as in excoriation [skin-picking] disorder; stereotypies, as in stereotypic movement disorder; ritualized eating behavior, as in eating disorders; preoccupation with substances or gambling, as in substance-related and addictive disorders; preoccupation with having an illness, as in illness anxiety disorder; sexual urges or fantasies, as in paraphilic disorders; impulses, as in disruptive, impulse-control, and conduct disorders; guilty ruminations, as in major depressive disorder; thought insertion or delusional preoccupations, as in schizophrenia spectrum and other psychotic disorders; or repetitive patterns of behavior, as in autism spectrum disorder).

Specify if:

- **With good or fair insight:** The individual recognizes that obsessive-compulsive disorder beliefs are definitely or probably not true or that they may or may not be true.

- **With poor insight:** The individual thinks obsessive-compulsive disorder beliefs are probably true.

- **With absent insight/delusional beliefs:** The individual is completely convinced that obsessive-compulsive disorder beliefs are true.

(Reprinted with permission from the *Diagnostic and Statistical Manual of Mental Disorders, Fifth Edition,* © 2013. American Psychiatric Association.)

TABLE 8.5 ⌇ Diagnostic Criteria for Narcissistic Personality Disorder

A pervasive pattern of grandiosity (in fantasy or behavior), need for admiration, and lack of empathy, beginning by early adulthood and present in a variety of contexts, as indicated by five (or more) of the following:

1. Has a grandiose sense of self-importance (e.g., exaggerates achievements and talents, expects to be recognized as superior without commensurate achievements).

2. Is preoccupied with fantasies of unlimited success, power, brilliance, beauty, or ideal love .

3. Believes that he or she is "special" and unique and can only be understood by, or should associate with, other special or high-status people (or institutions).

4. Requires excessive admiration.

5. Has a sense of entitlement, i.e., unreasonable expectations of especially favorable treatment or automatic compliance with his or her expectations.

6. Is interpersonally exploitative, i.e., takes advantage of others to achieve his or her own ends.

7. Lacks empathy: is unwilling to recognize or identify with the feelings and needs of others.

8. Is often envious of others or believes that others are envious of him or her.

9. Shows arrogant, haughty behaviors or attitudes.

(Reprinted with permission from the *Diagnostic and Statistical Manual of Mental Disorders, Fifth Edition,* © 2013. American Psychiatric Association.)

TABLE 8.6 ⌇ Diagnostic Criteria for Separation Anxiety Disorder

A. Developmentally inappropriate and excessive fear or anxiety concerning separation from those to whom the individual is attached, as evidenced by at least three of the following:

1. Recurrent excessive distress when anticipating or experiencing separation from home or from major attachment figures.

2. Persistent and excessive worry about losing major attachment figures or about possible harm to them, such as illness, injury, disasters, or death.

3. Persistent and excessive worry about experiencing an untoward event (e.g., getting lost, being kidnapped, having an accident, becoming ill) that causes separation from a major attachment figure.

4. Persistent reluctance or refusal to go out, away from home, to school, to work, or elsewhere because of fear of separation.

5. Persistent and excessive fear of or reluctance about being alone or without major attachment figures at home or in other settings.

6. Persistent reluctance or refusal to sleep away from home or to go to sleep without being near a major attachment figure.

7. Repeated nightmares involving the theme of separation.

TABLE 8.6  (*continued*)

8. Repeated complaints of physical symptoms (e.g., headaches, stomachaches, nausea, vomiting) when separation from major attachment figures occurs or is anticipated.

B. The fear, anxiety, or avoidance is persistent, lasting at least 4 weeks in children and adolescents and typically 6 months or more in adults.

C. The disturbance causes clinically significant distress or impairment in social, academic, occupational, or other important areas of functioning.

D. The disturbance is not better explained by another mental disorder, such as refusing to leave home because of excessive resistance to change in autism spectrum disorder; delusions or hallucinations concerning separation in psychotic disorders; refusal to go outside without a trusted companion in agoraphobia; worries about ill health or other harm befalling significant others in generalized anxiety disorder; or concerns about having an illness in illness anxiety disorder.

(Reprinted with permission from the *Diagnostic and Statistical Manual of Mental Disorders, Fifth Edition,* © 2013. American Psychiatric Association.)

TABLE 8.7  Diagnostic Criteria for Gender Dysphoria in Children

A. A marked incongruence between one's experienced/expressed gender and assigned gender, of at least 6 months' duration, as manifested by at least six of the following (one of which must be Criterion A1):

1. A strong desire to be of the other gender or an insistence that one is the other gender (or some alternative gender different from one's assigned gender).

2. In boys (assigned gender), a strong preference for cross-dressing or simulating female attire; or in girls (assigned gender), a strong preference for wearing only typical masculine clothing and a strong resistance to the wearing of typical feminine clothing.

3. A strong preference for cross-gender roles in make-believe play or fantasy play.

4. A strong preference for the toys, games, or activities stereotypically used or engaged in by the other gender.

5. A strong preference for playmates of the other gender.

6. In boys (assigned gender), a strong rejection of typically masculine toys, games, and activities and a strong avoidance of rough-and-tumble play; or in girls (assigned gender), a strong rejection of typically feminine toys, games, and activities.

7. A strong dislike of one's sexual anatomy.

8. A strong desire for the primary and/or secondary sex characteristics that match one's experienced gender.

The condition is associated with clinically significant distress or impairment in social, school, or other important areas of functioning

(Reprinted with permission from the *Diagnostic and Statistical Manual of Mental Disorders, Fifth Edition,* © 2013. American Psychiatric Association.)

Chapter 9 Notes

1. A sleepy waiter in Chapter 19 of *David Copperfield* exhibited symptoms of restless leg syndrome. New to the DSM-5, restless leg syndrome has been designated a separate entity and been removed from sleep disorders "not otherwise specified."

Chapter 11 Notes

1. I have quoted Falstaff's comment from the end of Scene Two of the First Act of Henry IV, Part 2 "a pox of this gout, or a gout of this pox, for the one or the other plays the rogue with my great toe" to many patients I have seen with gout. Whether the patients knew Shakespeare well or not, all have agreed that Falstaff well characterized and summarized their predicament.

2. Shakespeare's *Hamlet* is famous for containing a play-within-a-play (Act 3, Scene 2). Act V, Scene 1 of *Macbeth* may suggest that plays-within-a-play are more common that typically thought. Given that Shakespeare was the ultimate man of the theater perhaps this shouldn't be surprising. Another example is Malvolio's soliloquy in Act 2, Scene 5 of *Twelfth Night* that is observed and commented about (from inside a tree) by Sir Toby Belch, Sir Andrew and Fabian. It would be interesting to see if most (or even all?!) of Shakespeare's plays feature an embedded performance.

3. Pope and colleagues (2007) find our *Macbeth* example in the class of a work by Quintus Smyrnaeus (4th Century BCE) (*The Fall of Troy* [www.gutenberg.org/dirs/etext96/ftroy10.txt], see Book XIV, lines 160ff.) and Charlotte Smith (1788).

    In book fourteen of his Fall of Troy Menelaus tells Helen "No more remember past griefs: seal them up | Hid in thine heart. Let all be locked within | The dim dark mansion of forgetfulness. | What profits it to call ill deeds to mind?"

    In her Elegiac Sonnet number 40 Smith writes "Can the soft lustre of the sleeping main, | Yon radiant heaven, or all creation's charms, | Erase the written troubles of the brain, | Which Memory tortures, and which Guilt alarms?"

    Immediately, it is most interesting to see that *Macbeth* is the source of Smith's sonnet. We also see that Shakespeare is quite possibly the source of Victorian writers (and others) who suggested the possibility of repressed memories. Indeed, Macbeth is in fact much different than Smymaeus and Smith where there is the wish to forget unhappy memories but (1) it tends to a large general set of memories rather than the possibility Shakespeare suggests of removing a single memory, (2) crucially, in Smymaeus it is hoped that the heart can somehow erase

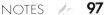

unpleasant memories, and in Smith, Nature is called upon to do so. Shakespeare appreciates that a neurologic process is necessary for this and that it appears to take medical/scientific intervention to do so.

Chapter 12 Notes

1. Poe's 1841 "Murders in the Rue Morgue" is the first modern detective story complete with "Sherlockian" sleuth C. Auguste Dupin, though Das Fräulein von Scuderi (1819) by German writer and music and literary critic E. T. A. Hoffmann and Zadig (1747) by the French philosopher Voltaire feature detective work. In looking for more proximal influences on Poe by looking at shared text and obscure references Kevin Hayes (2010, 2011) has found that Poe read the "Bibliophilist, which was written by English dandy and diarist Thomas Raikes. (Dickens included the story in the June 1838 Bentley's *Miscellany* and "The Scrap-Stall" (1838) by British novelist Catherine Grace Frances Gore. Both of these stories have elements of the modern procedural. It would be interesting to have a television series of "before Holmes" or "before Poe" mysteries!

   I was somewhat more surprised to come across a 1973 *New England Journal of Medicine article* (Sandler, 1973) which well summarizes the case that Poe derived the internal line rhyme and meter for his great poem *The Raven* (1845) from Chivers' 1842 *To Allegra Florence in Heaven*. Further, the refrain "Nevermore" in *The Raven* may well be derived from Chivers' 1839 *Lament on the Death of My Mother*, and Poe's poem *The Bells* (1849) from Chivers' 1845 *A Mother's Lament on the Death of Her Child*. Thomas Holley Chivers was a physician from Georgia who left the practice of clinical medicine in 1831 to pursue poetry. Chivers was a correspondent of Poe's and his highly imaginative and lyrical poems were widely published in his lifetime, read to classes at Harvard by James Russell Lowell and were influential not only with Poe but with other writers such as Rudyard Kipling.

Chapter 13 Notes

1. When reading the *Iliad* and *Odyssey*—the oldest written documents of a culture—and paying attention to the facts, or what has been written as being already known, the reader can catch a glimpse of what the time *before* the texts were written was like. Along with Heracles and his labors—which were clearly well known to Homer's readers—here are some other examples of references to Greek pre-Epic culture: The women warriors of Amazonia are mentioned *The Iliad* Book 3. *The Iliad* (Book 7, line 468 and Book 23, line 746) mentions Jason without need for further elaboration. This indicates that Jason's quest as captain of the ship Argo leading heroes including Heracles to the Black Sea coast to

retrive the Golden Fleece was a story well-known already to Homer's readers. *The Odyssey* Book 4, line 130 mentions Alkandre's travels to Egypt. Herodatus in his *Histories* appreciates the travels of this long famed traveler. In Book 8, line 224 the bowman Eurytos is mentioned. Eurytos was so proud of his skill in archery, he challenged Apollo to a contest. Apollo then killed him in anger. Book 10 of the *Odyssey* line 496 mentions the blind Thebean seer Theiresias in a manner indicating that Theirsias was a figure already known to readers of the *Odyssey*.

An interesting recurring story in *The Iliad* (first mentioned in Book 10, line 17) and *The Odyssey* is that of Neleus, a predecessor of Nestor as king of Pylos. As it is, Nestor is the wise old man of the *Iliad* and *Odyssey*. Nestor seems at least two generations older than other characters in the epics. Neleus is mentioned in the *Odyssey* Book 3, lines 406–409, Book 11, line 250 and lines 282–284 which describes how Neleus wooed and married the lovely Khloris. The exploits of Neleus are also mentioned in Book 15 lines 221–230.

References

Abdul-Hamid, W. K., and Hughes, J. H. 2014. Nothing new under the sun: post-traumatic stress disorders in the ancient world. *Early Sci Med* 19: 549–557.

Adler, J. J. 1983. Did Falstaff have the sleep-apnea syndrome? *New England Journal of Medicine* 308: 404.

Altschuler, E. L. 1999. Helpful portrayals of obsessive-compulsive disorder. *Lancet* 354: 871.

Altschuler, E. L. 2001. Art. *Lancet* 357: 895.

Altschuler, E. L. 2001. One of the oldest cases of schizophrenia in Gogol's *Diary of a Madman*. *BMJ* 323: 1475–1477.

Altschuler, E. L. 2003. Hereditary somnambulism in Dracula. *J R Soc Med.* 96: 51–52.

Altschuler, E. L. 2003. Informed consent in an Edgar Allan Poe tale. *Lancet* 362: 1504.

Altschuler, E. L. 2004. Prescient description of frontal lobe syndrome in an Edgar Allan Poe tale. *Lancet* 363: 902.

Altschuler, E. L. 2008. Brain contusion/sudden cardiopulmonary arrest syndrome in *A Painful Case* from James Joyce's Dubliners. *S Afr Med J* 98: 442.

Altschuler, E. L. 2013. Asperger's in the Holmes Family. *J Autism Dev Disord* 43: 2238–2239.

Altschuler, E. L. 2016. PTSD induced by the trauma of subordinates: The Robert Gates syndrome. *Occupational Medicine* 66: 182.

Altschuler, E. L., and Augenstein, S. 2012. The earliest description of the frontal lobe syndrome in an Edgar Allan Poe tale. *Brain Inj* 26: 1403–1404.

Altschuler, E. L., and Wright, D. 2000. Dr. Jekyll and Mr. Hyde: A primer on substance dependence. *Am J Psychiatry* 157: 484.

Altschuler, E. L., Haroun, A., Ho, B., and Weiner, A. 2001. Did Samson have antisocial personality disorder? *Archives of General Psychiatry* 58: 202–203.

Altschuler, E. L., Haroun, A., Ho, B., and Weiner, A. 2001. Did Samson have antisocial personality disorder? *Archives of General Psychiatry* 59: 565–596.

Altschuler, E. L., Ramachandran, V. S., and Ravi, V. S. 2007. Verifiable cases of repressed memories. *Psychol Med* 37: 1067.

Anderson, S. W., Bechara, A., Damasio, H., Tranel, D., and Damasio, A. R. 1999. Impairment of social and moral behavior related to early damage in human prefrontal cortex. *Nat Neurosci* 2: 1032–1037.

Aruz, J., Farkas, A., Alekseev, A., and Korolkova, E. (eds). 2000. *The golden deer of Eurasia: Scythian and Sarmatian treasures from the Russian steppes*. The State Hermitage, Saint Petersburg, and the Archaeological Museum. Metropolitan Museum of Art, NY.

Asperger, H. 1944. Die "Autistischen Psychopathen" im Kindes-alter. *Archiv für psychiatrie und nervenkrankheiten* 117: 76–136.

Auster, S. 1999. Attention deficit disorder. *Pediatrics* 104: 1419.

Benitez, R. M. 1996. A 39-year-old man with mental status change. *Md Med J* 45: 765–769.

Bentley, S. 2005. Short history of PTSD: From Thermopylae to Hue soldiers have always had a disturbing reaction to war. *Vietnam Veterans of America: The Veteran*. http://www.vva.org/archive/TheVeteran/2005_03/feature_HistoryPTSD.htm

Brain, R. 1955. Dickensian diagnoses. *BMJ* 1553–1556.

Brugger, P., Agosti, R., Regard, M., Wieser, H. G., and Landis, T. 1994. Heautoscopy, epilepsy, and suicide. *J Neurol Neurosurg Psychiatry* 57: 838–839.

Burwell, C. S., Robin, E. D., Whaley, R. D., et al. 1956. Extreme obesity associated with alveolar hypoventilation: A Pickwickian syndrome. *Am J Med* 21: 811–818.

Casey, R. L. 1967. Shakespeare and Elizabethan surgery. *Surg Gynecol Obstet* 124: 1324.

Čatipović, B. 2004. Myostatin mutation associated with gross muscle hypertrophy in a child. *N Engl J Med* 351: 1030.

Clawson, A. H., Jurbergs, N., Lindwall, J., and Phipps, S. 2013. Concordance of parent proxy report and child self-report of posttraumatic stress in children with cancer and healthy children: influence of parental posttraumatic stress. *Psycho-Oncology* 22: 2593–2600.

Cosman, B. C. 1998. All's Well That Ends Well: Shakespeare's treatment of anal fistula. *Dis Colon Rectum* 41: 914–924.

Cosnett, J. E. 1991. Dickens, dystonia and dyskinesia. *J Neurol Neurosurg Psychiatry* 54: 184.

Cosnett, J. E. 1992. Charles Dickens: observer of sleep and its disorders. *Sleep* 15: 264–247.

Cotterill, J. A. 1972. Shakespeare on the skin. *Br J Dermatol* 86: 533–542.

Cybulska, E. 1998. Senile squalor: Plyushkin's not diogenes syndrome. *Psychiatric Bulletin* 22: 319–320.

Da Costa, J. M. 1871. On Irritable Heart: A Clinical Study of a Form of Functional Cardiac Disorder and its Consequences. *American Journal of the Medical Sciences* 61: 17–52.

Davis, E., Hayes, M., and Dirman, B. H. 1942. Somnambulism. *Lancet* i: 186.

Dickens, C., and Collins, W. 1857. The lazy tour of two idle apprentices. In: *No thoroughfare and other stories*. Stroud: Alan Sutton; 1990. p 128–227.

Donvan J., and Zucker, C. 2016. The Early History of Autism in America. *Smithsonian Magazine* January.

Down, J. L. 1864. Polysarcia and its treatment. *London Hosp Rep* 1: 97–103.

Doyle, A. C. 1893. The adventure of the Greek interpreter in The Memoirs of Sherlock Holmes (London). http://en.wikisource.org/ wiki/The_Greek_Interpreter.

Doyle, A. C. 1917. The adventure of the Bruce-Partington plans, Part I. In *His Last Bow* (London). http://en.wikisource.org/wiki/The_ Adventure_of_the_Bruce-Partington_Plans.

Dvorak, S. 1966. Unexpected meteor shower from Lyra. *Sky & Telescope* 32: 237.

Dykens, E. M. 2002. Are jigsaw puzzle skills 'spared' in persons with Prader-Willi syndrome? *J Child Psychol Psychiatry* 43: 343–352.

Ehrlich, G. E. 1967. Shakespeare's rheumatology. *Ann Rheum Dis* 26: 562–563.

Elwin, M. 1950. *The Strange Case of Robert Louis Stevenson.* Macdonald, London.

Erichsen, J. E. 1867. *On Railway and Other Injuries of the Nervous System.* Henry C. Lea, Philadelphia.

Estanol, B. V., and Marin, O. S. 1975. Cardiac arrythmias and sudden death in subarachnoid hemorrhage. *Stroke* 6: 382–386.

Ezekowitz, R. A. 1998. Genetic heterogeneity of mannose-binding proteins: The Jekyll and Hyde of innate immunity? *Am J Hum Genet* 62: 6–9.

Ezra, M. G. 2001. Earliest evidence of post-traumatic stress? *Br J Psychiatry* 179: 467.

Fanger, D. 1979. *The creation of Nikolai Gogol.* Belknap Press, Cambridge, MA.

Fluckiger-Hawker, E. 1999. *Urnamma of Ur in Sumerian Literary Tradition.* University Press Fribourg, Guttingen.

Fogan, L. 1989. The neurology in Shakespeare. *Arch Neurol* 46: 922–924.

Gates, R. M. 2014. *Duty* Vintage, New York.

Gault, J. E. 1965. Did Winnie the Pooh have spontaneous functional hypoglycaemia? *Med J Aust.* 32: 942–943.

Gilles de la Tourette, G. 1885. Etude sur une affection nerveuse caracterisee par de l'incoordination motrice accompagnee d'echolalie et de coprolalie. *Archives de Neurologie* 9: 19–42, 158–200.

Gogol, N. V., and Maguire, R. A. 2004. *Dead souls: A poem.* Penguin, London.

Gomez-Alonso, J. 1998. A possible explanation for the vampire legend. *Neurology* 51: 856–859.

Gould, S. J. 1980. "A Biological Homage to Mickey Mouse" in *The Panda's Thumb.* W.W. Norton & Company.

Grinker, R. R., and Spiegel, J. P. 1945 *Men Under Stress.* Blakiston, Philadelphia.

Hare, E. 1988. Schizophrenia as a recent disease. *British Journal of Psychiatry* 153: 521–531.

Harlow, J. M. 1848. Passage of an iron rod through the head. *Boston Med Surg J* 39: 389–393.

Haslam, J. 1798. *Observations on Insanity.* Rivington, London.

Haslam, J. 1809. *Observations on melancholy and madness.* Callow, London.

Hayes, K. J. 2011. Mrs Gore and "The Murders at the Rue Morgue." *Notes and Queries* 58: 85–87.

Hayes, K. J., 2010. Another source for the Fall of the House of Usher. *Notes and Queries* 57: 214–216.

Heick, A. 1992. Prince Dracula, rabies, and the vampire legend. *Ann Intern Med* 117: 172–173.

Hocke, V., and Schmidtke, A. 1998. "Multiple personality disorder" in childhood and adolescence. *Z Kinder Jugendpsychiatr Psychother* 26: 273–284.

Hoffmann, H. 1935. Slovenly Peter (Der Struwwelpeter, translated into English jingles from the original German of Dr Heinrich Hoffmann by Mark Twain, with Dr. Hoffmann's illustrations adapted from the rare first edition by Fritz Kredel). Marchbanks Press, New York.

Hogarth, D. J. 1916. http://www.gutenberg.org/files/1081/1081-h/1081-h.htm.

http://en.wikipedia.org/wiki/Horace_Vernet

http://fmso.leavenworth.army.mil/Collaboration/international/Sri%20Lanka/PTSD.pdf

http://www.cmaj.ca/content/163/12/1557.full/reply#cmaj_el_78

https://www.nichd.nih.gov/health/topics/autism/conditioninfo/Pages/at-risk.aspx

Huber, T. J., and te Wildt, B. T. 2005. Charles Dickens' A Tale of Two Cities: A case report of posstraumatic stress disorder. *Psychopathology* 38: 334–337.

Insanity—illustrated by histories of distinguished men, and by the writings of poets and novelists. 1844. *American Journal of Insanity* 1: 9–46. (Articles in the early issues of the journals did not list authors.)

Itard, J. M. G. 1825. Mémoire sur quelques functions involontaires des appareils de la locomotion, de la préhension et de la voix. *Arch Gen Med* 8: 385–407.

Jacoby, N. M. 1992. Krook's dyslexia. *Lancet* 340: 1521–1522.

Jayatunge, R. M. 2010. *Post-Traumatic Stress Disorder (PTSD): A Malady Shared by East and West: A Sri Lankan Look at Combat Stress and Trauma.*

Kales, A., Soldatos, C. R., Boxler, E. O., et al. 1980. Hereditary factors in sleepwalking and night terrors. *Br J Psychiatry* 137: 111–118.

Kanner, L. 1943. Autistic disturbances of affective contact. *Nerv Child* 2: 217–250.

Kast, R. E., and Altschuler, E. L. 2008. The earliest example of the hyperactivity subtype of attention deficit hyperactivity disorder (ADHD) in Jan Steen's 'The Village School' (c. 1670). *S Afr Med J* 98: 594–595.

Katragadda, S., and Schubiner, H. 2007. ADHD in children, adolescents, and adults. *Prim Care* 34: 317–341.

Kaufmann, F. 1916. Die planmäBige Heilung komplizierter psychogener Bewegungsstörungen bei Soldaten in einer Sitzung. In: *Feldärtz Beilage Münch Med Wochenschr* 63: 802.

Knoch, D., Gianotti, L. R, Mohr, C., and Brugger, P. 2005. Synesthesia: When colors count. *Cogn Brain Res* 25: 372–374.

Kohl, F. 1999. The beginning of Emil Kraepelin's classification of psychoses. A historical-methodological reflection on the occasion of the 100th anniversary of his "Heidelberg Address" 27 November 1898 on "nosologic dichotomy" of endogenous psychoses. *Psychiatr Prax* 26: 105–111.

Larner, A. J. 2002. Did Charles Dickens describe progressive supranuclear palsy in 1857? *Movement Disorders* 17: 832–833.

Mackinnon, R. A., and Yudofsky, S. C. 1986. *The Psychiatric Evaluation in Clinical Practice*, pp. 125–128. Lippincott, Philadelphia.

MacWilliam, J. A. 1889. Cardiac failure and sudden death. *British Medical Journal* i: 6–8.

Margolis, M. L. 2000. Brahms' lullaby revisited. Did the composer have obstructive sleep apnea? *Chest* 118: 210–213.

Milian, G. 1915. L'hypnose des batailles. *Paris Med.* 2: 265–270.

Milovanovic, A. V., and DiMaio, V. J. 1999. Death due to concussion and alcohol. *Am J Forensic Med Patho* 20: 6–9.

Mitchell, S. W. 1876. Some disorders of sleep. *Virginia Medical Monthly* 2: 769–781.

Myers, C. M. 1915. Contributions to the study of shell shock. *Lancet* 13: 316–320.

Number of the Insane and Idiotic, with brief notes of the lunatic asylums in the United States. 1844. *American Journal of Insanity* 1: 78–88. (Articles in the early issues of the journals did not list authors.)

Olson, D. W. 2014. *Celestial Sleuth,* pp. 345–349. Springer, New York.

Olson, D. W., and Olson, M. S. 2004. The June Lyrids and James Joyce's *Ulysses*. *Sky & Telescope* 108: 28–33.

Perkin, G. D. 1996. Disorders of gait. *J Neurol Neurosurg Psychiatry* 61: 199.

Pinel, P. 1801. *Traité médico-philosophique sur l'aliénation mentale.* J. A. Brosson, Paris

Pinel, P. 1809. *Traité médico-philosophique sur l'aliénation mentale* (2nd ed.). J. A. Brosson, Paris.

Pope Jr., H. G., et al. 2007. Is dissociative amnesia a culture-bound syndrome? Findings from a survey of historical Literature. *Psychological Medicine* 37: 225–233.

Pope-Hennessy, J. 1974. *Robert Louis Stevenson.* Jonathan Cape, London.

Prader, A., Labhart, A., Willi, H. 1956. Ein Syndrom von Adipositas, Kleinwuchs, Kryptorchismus und Oligophrenie nach Myatonieartigem Zustand im Neugeborenenalter. *Schweiz Med Wschr.* 86: 1260–1261.

Sacks, O. 2001. Henry Cavendish: An early case of Asperger's syndrome? *Neurology* 57: 1347.

Salmon, T. W. 1917. Care and treatment of mental disease and war neuroses (shell shock) in the British army. New York: War Work Committee of the National Committee for Mental Hygiene. OCLC 11539475.

Sandler, S. G. 1973. Thomas Holley Chivers, M.D. (1809–1858) and the origin of Edgar Allan Poe's *The Raven*. 289: 351–354.

Schuelke, M., Wagner, K. R., Stolz, L. E., et al. 2004. Myostatin mutation associated with gross muscle hypertrophy in a child. *N Engl J Med* 350: 2682–2688.

Schultz, M. 1971. The "Strange Case" of Robert Louis Stevenson. *JAMA* 216: 90–94.

Shay, J. 2013. Annotations adapted from those of clinical psychiatrist Jonathan Shay https://www.publicinsightnetwork.org/2013/05/28/a-shakespearean-view-of-ptsd/

Shea, S. E., Gordon, K., Hawkins, A., Kawchuk, J., and Smith, D. 2000. Pathology in the Hundred Acres Wood: A neurodevelopmental perspective on A. A. Milne. *CAMJ* 163: 1557–1559.

Smith, C. 1993. Elegiac Sonnnet: 40. In *The Poems of Charlotte Smith* (ed. S. Curran). Oxford University Press.

Steele J. C., Richardson J. C., and Olszewski J. 1964. Progressive supranuclear palsy. A heterogenous degeneration involving the brain stem, basal ganglia and cerebellum with vertical gaze and pseudobulbar palsy, nuchal dystonia and dementia. *Arch Neurol.* 10: 333–359.

Stevenson, R. L. 1981. *The Strange Case of Dr. Jekyll and Mr. Hyde* (1886). Bantam Books, New York.

Still, G. 1902. The Goulstonian Lectures on some abnormal psychical conditions in children: Lecture I [II, III]. *Lancet* 1: 1008–1012; 1077–1082; 1163–1168.

Summerskill, W. H. J. 1955. Augecheek's disease. *Lancet* ii: 288.

Tabaaa, M. A., Ramirez-Lassepas, M., and Snyder, B. D. 1987. Aneurysmal subarachnoid hemorrhage presenting as cardiopulmonary arrest. *Archives of Internal Medicine* 147: 1661–1662.

Thome, J., and Jacobs, K. A. 2004. Attention deficit hyperactivity disorder (ADHD) in a 19th century children's book. *Eur Psychiatry* 19: 303–306.

Whitehead, F. A., Liese, B. S., and O'Dell, M. L. 1990. Melville's "Bartleby the Scrivener": A case study. *N Y State J Med* 90: 17–22.

Yudofsky, S. C., and Silver, J. M. 1987. Aggressive behavior in patients with neuropsychiatric disorders. *Psychiatric Annals* 17: 367–370.

Zekman, T. N., and Davis, E. H. 1969. Shakespeare's ophthalmologic vocabulary and concepts. *Am J Ophthalmol* 68: 1–9.

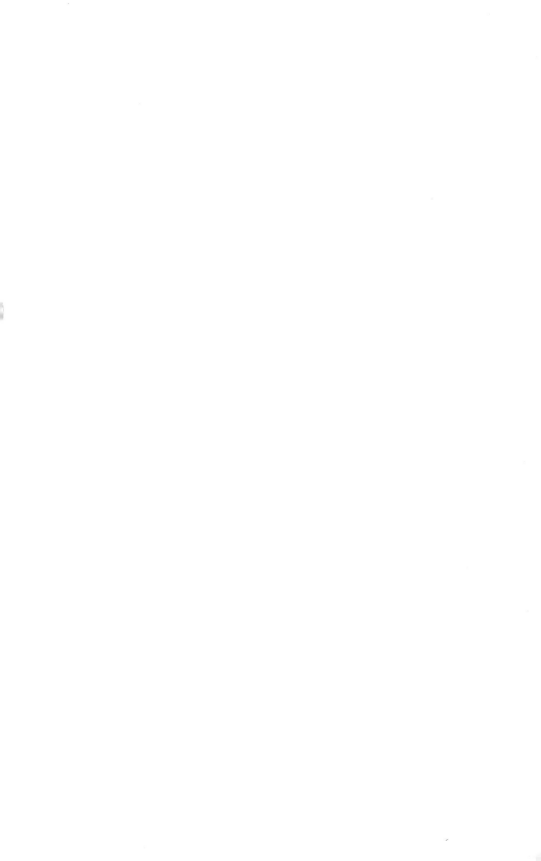